TRAEGER GRILL
BIBLE

TRAEGER RECIPES WITH REAL BBQ FLAVOUR. IMPRESS YOUR GUESTS!

FIRE ACADEMY 2.0

INTRODUCTION

The Traeger grill is extremely popular these days. It is one of the most convenient and versatile cookers on the market. With this cooking device, you don't have to stand over a fire and cook. You get a consistent temperature and perfectly cooked food every time. With a Traeger grill, you don't have to worry about fuel, temperature control, or flare-ups. Instead, you can focus on the most important thing: creating a spectacular meal. Often beginners shy away from grills because they think they are unsafe and too complicated to use. However, with the Traeger grill, the only thing you need is the right guide.

This Traeger grill cookbook will teach you all the tricks and techniques you need to become a grill master. Use this smoker to cook perfect beef, pork, lamb, chicken, turkey, fish, and seafood every time. This Traeger grill guide for beginners presents a complete cookbook with 300 tasty recipes to utilize your Traeger grill to its full potential. With this grill, you can cook the best cuts of meats, ribs, burgers, sausages, side dishes, snacks, and even desserts. This book includes a comprehensive collection of smoke beef, pork, lamb, poultry, game, fish, and seafood, side dishes, snacks, and desserts with easy step-by-step explanations. This cookbook will show you that you can cook anything on a Traeger.

Whether you are a beginner or an experienced griller, whether you prefer grilling, smoking, baking, direct cooking, or barbecuing, this book got you covered. All the recipes included in this book are delicious and tasty. Cook these mouthwatering meals for your family and friends, and they will love them. This grilling guide is perfect for beginners as long as experienced grill masters who want to expand their cooking assortment.

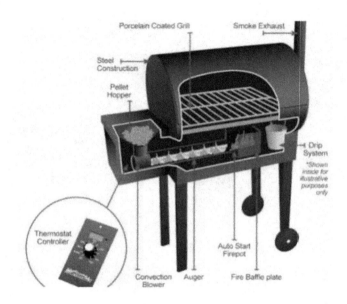

Traeger Grill and Smoker

Pellet grills are outdoor cookers that utilize modern technologies to ignite all-natural hardwood pellets as a fuel source for heating and cooking your food. Most pellet grills have temperature ranges near 200F to 500F, which is an ample range to handle hot searing grill jobs as well as low and slow smoking.

An important note about your pellet grill – it does not cook with direct heat. Pellet grills have a deflector plate that distributes heat around the cooking chamber, where air and heat flow similar to a convection oven. This is exactly why it is possible to also bake and roast on your pellet grill.

Why choose Traeger grill

1. Better flavor. The Traeger grill uses all-natural wood, so food comes out better-tasting compared to when you cook them in a gas or charcoal grill.
2. No flare-ups: No flare-ups mean that food is cooked evenly on all sides. This is made possible by using indirect heat. Because there are no flare-ups, you can smoke and bake without some areas or sides of your food burning.
3. Mechanical parts are well designed and protected.
4. Exceptional temperature control.
5. Built-in Wi-Fi: So you can set up Traeger Grills even if you are not physically present in front of the grills.
6. Environmentally friendly

Different types of Traeger Grill

1. Gas grills: These grills tend to mostly run on natural gas.
2. Charcoal grills: They tend to mostly make use of charcoal briquettes as the source of fuel.
3. Electric grills: These grills use the electric source as a means to get fired up.

Smoking Meat Basic Tips

1. Smoking food needs a low heat and keeps it low for a few hours allowing the smoke to penetrate through the meats. The procedure is very simple: pile the coals over the bottom, then add the smoking wood and put the meat onto the grill right into the opposite side of

the coals you use. Add more coal from time to time to maintain the same temperature.

2. Smoking meat needs patience. So you need to be patient when using Traeger grill to cook meats.

3. Dry or wet smoking process. The wet smoking process includes a pan filled with water and coals that can create a smoky atmosphere that will help moisturize the meat. You can also use fruit juice or any other type of equipment to add extra flavors.

4. Using a rub is substantial in any smoking process. Use a rub mixture over your meat right before you start smoking.

5. Choose the right woold. In order to smoke meat properly, you should carefully choose the wood you are going to use.

What are pellets

Traeger wood pellet grills are electric grills that use wood pellets as their fuel source. The specially designed wood pellets can also be used as flavor enhancers to give food an excellent smoky taste. Traeger woold pellet grill and smoker does not require constant monitoring and can be left to regulate itself while cooking.

Pellet grills are outdoor cookers that utilize modern technologies to ignite all-natural hardwood pellets as a fuel source for heating and cooking your food.

Types of Pellets

Traeger offers a variety of wood pellets to use in their grills. All are made from 100 percent natural, food-grade Hardwood that will burn clean and provide an optimal wood-fired flavor.

PELLET TYPE	DESCRIPTION	RECOMMENDED COOKS
Hickory	Strong smoke flavor	Beef and pork
Mesquite	Strong smoke flavor	Beef and seafood
Apple	Mild, dense fruit flavor, sweet smoke and most common of fruitwoods	Pork, chicken, sides, and desserts
Cherry	Subtly sweet fruity flavor provides great color	Pork, chicken, seafood, and desserts
Oak	Medium to heavy smoke flavor, slightly nutty	Beef
Alder	Light smoke flavor, mild wood	Seafood, vegetables, and baked items
Pecan	Medium smoke flavor, sweet and mild flavor	Poultry, pork, vegetables, and desserts

Maple	Mild, sweet flavor	Poultry, seafood, and vegetables

Setting up the grill for smoking

- o Soak wood chips in a big bowl of water for at least 1 hour, and soak aromatic twigs for about 30 minutes.
- o Drain and remove excess water before adding soaked wood to the flames
- o Use long-handled tongs to position hot ash-covered coals around a foil pan that is filled with 1-inch of water.
- o Add coals with pre-soaked chunks, chips, and/or aromatics
- o Check food, temperature as well as water pan once per hour, adjusting as required.
- o Do not add additional wood during the last half of smoking time on Charcoal or a vertical smoker.
- o Make wood chips last longer and avoid burning by bundling wet wood chips in a foil packet with holes. Place the packet directly on the coals.

Top tips for searing on a grill

1. Ensure that the grill is clean. Food will stick to a dirty grill.

2. For even hotter grates, invest in cast iron grill grates

3. Get a hot surface for cooking 450F or more.

4. Lay the meat gently on the grates. Depending on the size of the meat and type, searing time varies, but you will usually want to sear for 3 to 5 minutes on each side.

5. Don't touch it before it is time to flip.

More tips

1. Reverse sear: Traeger pellet grill is perfect for reverse searing, which is perfect for foods like steak.

2. An oven: You can use it as an oven

3. Frozen meat: Put frozen meat directly at low temperature.

4. Use the upper rack: Using the upper rack increases the amount of food that can be cooked all at once.

Selecting Meat for Smoking

Choose the type of meat that tastes good with a smoky flavor. Following meat goes well for smoking.

o   Beef: ribs, brisket, and corned beef.

o   Pork: spare ribs, roast, shoulder, and ham.

o   Poultry: whole chicken, a whole turkey, and big game hens.

o   Seafood: Salmon, scallops, trout, and lobster.

Cleaning and maintenance of Traeger Grill

1. Clean the Smoke Exhaust with warm, soapy water or a biodegradable degreaser. Scrape accumulated creosote with a wooden or any other non-metallic tool.

2. Inspect the Grease Drain, Grease Drain Tube, and Grease Bucket for grease build-up. Clean regularly with soapy water and a soft brush or wipe with paper towels and rags. Lining a grease bucket with aluminum foil will make clean-up easier.

3. Clean Steel construction with warm, soapy water and rags to remove grease. Do not use abrasive materials to scrub, or it will peel off the non-stick surface.

4. Clean Porcelain grill while after every meal, while warm. Do this with a long-handled cleaning brush to prevent burns and injuries.

5. Remove ash accumulated inside and around Firepot. Sweep ash with a whisk broom or metal fireplace shovel.

Remember, do these activities when the grill is cold and disconnected from a power source.

Requested Smoker Control Settings	Suggested Thermostat Settings
Smoke	150-180°F (also smoke on Traeger Grill)
Medium	225-275°F
High	350-400°F

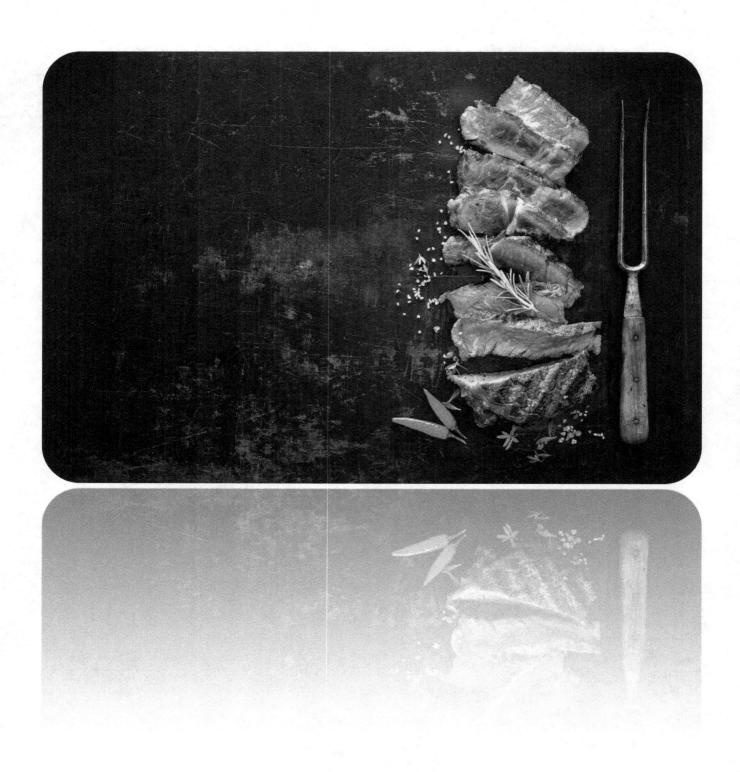

1. Beef Roast

Prep Time: 15 minutes | Cooking Time: 3 ½ hours | Temperature: 500F|

Servings: 6

Ingredients:

- 1 beef top round of about 3 to 3-1/2 sirloin tip roast or rump
- 3 tbsp. of extra-virgin olive oil
- As needed of Traeger Prime Rib Rub
- 2 cups of beef broth
- 1 large peeled and cut into pieces of 1-inch russet potato
- 2 carrots, peeled and cut into 1-inch pieces
- 2 cut into pieces of 1 inch of celery stalks
- 1 small onion, chopped into pieces of 1 inch each
- 2 sprigs of thyme

Directions:

1. Run the beef roast on all sides with oil and place over a rack into a roasting pan with the fat side up.
2. Season very well with Traeger Prime Rib Rub. Then pour the beef broth into the bottom of the pan.
3. Preheat the Traeger to about 500F with the lid closed for 15 minutes.
4. Cook the roast for 25 to 30 minutes or until the outside is very well seared.
5. Lower the temperature to about 225F, then add in the vegetables.
6. Cover with foil and cook for 2 to 3 hours or until the internal temperature reaches about 135F (for medium-rare).

7. Add additional broth if needed.

8. Remove from the grill and rest for 10 minutes.

9. Slice and serve with vegetables.

NUTRITION:

Calories: 257|Fat: 16g| Carb: 0g| Protein: 26g

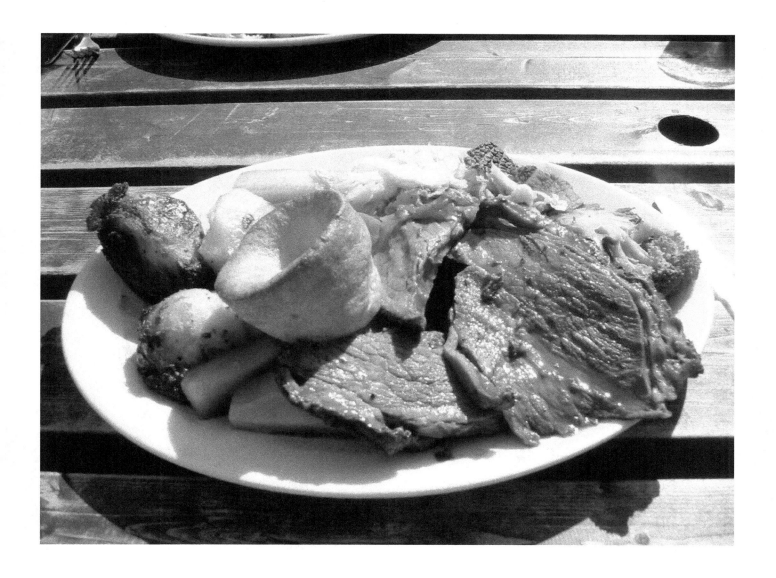

2. Beef Patties

Prep Time: 25 minutes | Cooking Time: 3 hours | Temperature: 325F | Servings: 6

Ingredients:

- 1 small, finely diced onion
- 3 large eggs, lightly beaten
- 2 egg yolks
- ¼ cup of milk
- ½ cup of ketchup
- ½ tsp. of salt
- ¼ tsp. of ground black pepper
- ½ tsp. of dry mustard
- ½ tsp. of onion powder
- ¼ tsp. of garlic powder
- 1 tsp. of dried parsley
- 1 tbsp. of minced garlic
- ½ cup of Panko breadcrumbs
- 1 sleeve of crushed saltine crackers
- 3 pounds of 85/15 ground beef

Directions:

1. Preheat the grill to 325F.
2. Finely dice the onion and mix in all the ingredients, except for the ground beef.
3. Stir everything to mix well. Then add the ground beef and mix well. Do not over mix.
4. Form small patties then set aside.
5. Carefully place the meat patties over the grill and cook for 10 to 15 minutes. Flip only once.
6. Place the BBQ sauce over the top and cook for 5 minutes more.
7. Put the cheese directly on top of the grill and cook for 10 to 15 minutes or until cheese melts.

8. Rest for 10 minutes. Serve | patties with buns.

NUTRITION:

Calories: 99|Fat: 5g| Carb: 11.3| Protein: 7g

3. Bacon-Swiss Cheesesteak Meatloaf

Prep Time: 15 minutes | Cooking Time: 2 hours | Temperature: 225F|
Servings: 8

Ingredients:

- 1 tbsp. oil
- 2 garlic cloves, finely chopped
- 1 medium onion, finely chopped
- 1 poblano chile, stemmed, seeded, and finely chopped
- 2 pounds extra-lean ground beef
- 2 tbsp. Montreal steak seasoning
- 1 tbsp. A.1. Steak Sauce
- ½ pound bacon, cooked and crumbled
- 2 cups shredded Swiss cheese
- 1 egg, beaten
- 2 cups breadcrumbs
- ½ cup Tiger Sauce

Directions:

1. Heat the oil on the stovetop in a pan.
2. Add garlic, onion, and poblano and sauté for 5 minutes.
3. Preheat the grill with the lid closed to 225F.
4. In a bowl, combine the sauteed vegetables, ground beef, steak seasoning, steak sauce, bacon, Swiss cheese, egg, and breadcrumbs.
5. Mix and shape into a loaf.
6. Put the meatloaf in a cast-iron skillet and place it on the grill.
7. Cook until the loaf reaches 165F.
8. Top the meatloaf with Tiger Sauce, and remove it from the grill.

9. Cool, slice, and serve.

NUTRITION:

Calories: 120|Fat: 2g| Carb: 0g| Protein: 23g

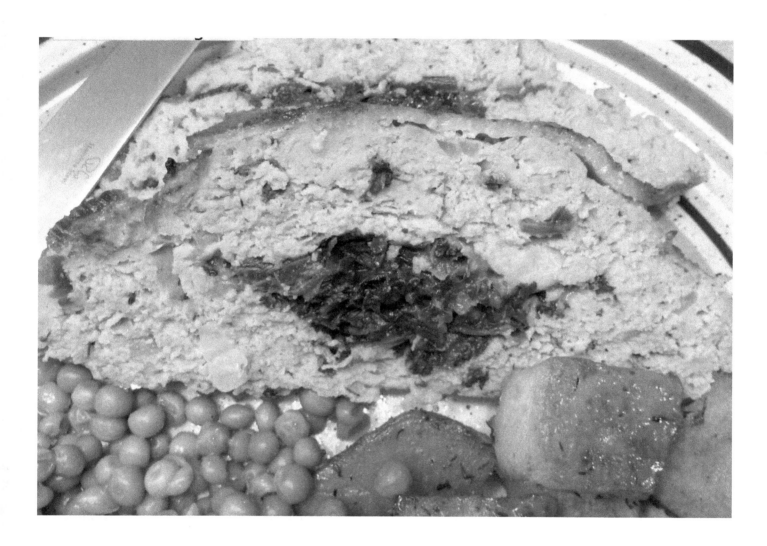

4. London Broil

Prep Time: 20 minutes | Cooking Time: 16 minutes | Temperature: 350F| Servings: 4

Ingredients:

- 1 (1½- to 2-pound) London broil or top round steak
- ¼ cup soy sauce
- 2 tbsp. white wine
- 2 tbsp. extra-virgin olive oil
- ¼ cup chopped scallions
- 2 tbsp. packed brown sugar
- 2 garlic cloves, minced
- 2 tsp. red pepper flakes
- 1 tsp. ground black pepper

Directions:

1. Pound the steak lightly with a meat mallet on both sides to break down its fibers and tenderize.
2. In a bowl, make the marinade by combining the soy sauce, white wine, olive oil, scallions, brown sugar, garlic, red pepper flakes, and black pepper.
3. Put the steak in a container with a lid and pour the marinade over the meat. Cover and refrigerate for 4 hours.
4. Preheat the grill with the lid closed to 350F.
5. Place the steak directly on the grill, close the lid, and smoke for 6 minutes.
6. Flip and smoke the lid closed for 6 to 10 minutes or until a meat thermometer inserted reads 130F for medium-rare.
7. Rest, slice, and serve.

NUTRITION:

Calories: 316|Fat: 3g| Carb: 0g| Protein: 54g

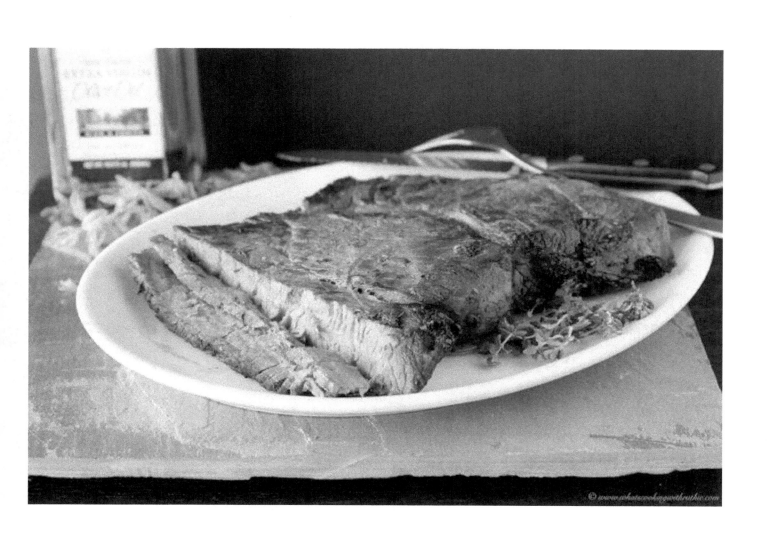

5. Beef Shoulder Clod

Prep Time: 10 minutes | Cooking Time: 16 hours | Temperature: 250F|
Servings: 20

Ingredients:

- ½ cup sea salt
- ½ cup ground black pepper
- 1 tbsp. red pepper flakes
- 1 tbsp. minced garlic
- 1 tbsp. cayenne pepper
- 1 tbsp. smoked paprika
- 1 (13- to 15-pound) beef shoulder clod

Directions:

1. Combine spices and generously apply them to the beef shoulder.
2. Preheat the grill with the lid closed to 250F.
3. Put the meat on the grill grate, and close the lid. Smoke for 12 to 16 hours, or until the meat reaches 195F. If necessary, cover the clod with foil toward the end of smoking to prevent over-browning.
4. Rest and serve.

NUTRITION:

Calories: 290|Fat: 22g| Carb: 0| Protein: 20g

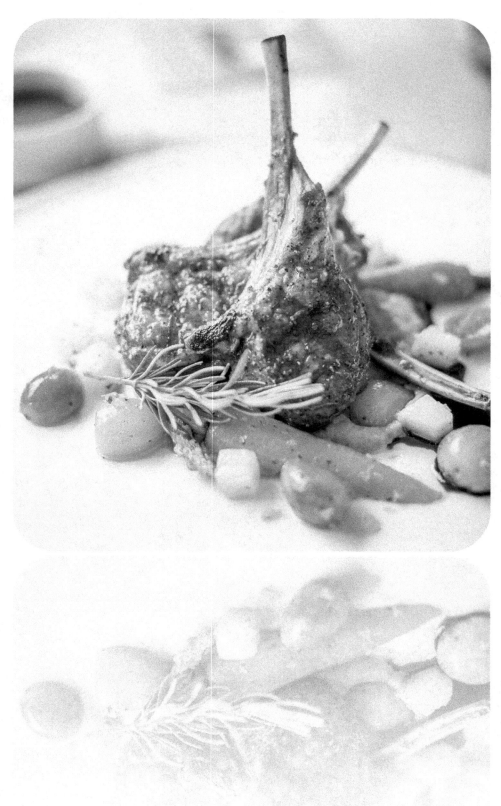

6. Braised Lamb Shank

Prep Time: 10 minutes | Cooking Time: 4 hours | Temperature: 500F|

Servings: 6

Ingredients:

- 6 whole lamb shanks
- Traeger Prime Rib Rub as needed
- 1 cup beef broth
- 1 cup red wine
- 4 sprig rosemary and thyme

Directions:

1. Season the lamb shanks with Traeger Prime Rib Rub.
2. Preheat the Traeger to 500F for 15 minutes with lid closed.
3. Place the lamb shanks directly on the grill grate and cook for 20 minutes or until the surface browns.
4. Transfer the shanks to a Dutch oven and pour in beef broth. Add the rosemary and thyme.
5. Place the Dutch oven on the grill gate and lower the temperature to 325F. Cook for 3 to 4 hours. Serve.

NUTRITION:

Calories: 532|Fat: 21.4g| Carb: 10.2g| Protein: 55.2g

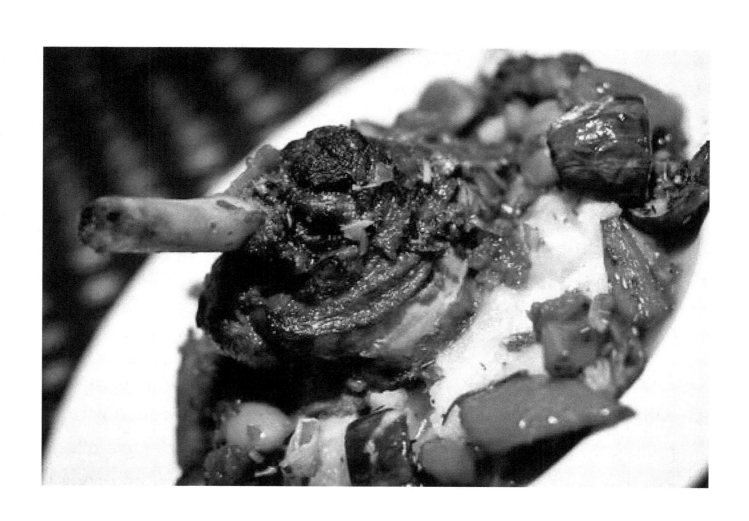

7. Smoked Lamb Leg with Salsa Verde

Prep Time: 10 minutes | Cooking Time: 3 hours | Temperature: 500F|
Servings: 6

Ingredients:

- 2 tbsp. oil
- 1 whole leg of lamb, fat trimmed and cut into chunks
- Salt to taste
- 6 cloves green garlic, unpeeled
- 1-pound tomatillos, husked and washed
- 1 small yellow onion, quartered
- 5 whole serrano chili peppers
- 1 tbsp. capers, drained
- ¼ cup cilantro, finely chopped
- ½ tsp. sugar
- 1 cup chicken broth
- 3 tbsp. lime juice, freshly squeezed

Directions:

1. Preheat the Traeger to 500F with the lid closed for 15 minutes.
2. Place a Dutch oven on the grill grate and add oil.
3. Put the lamb in the Dutch oven and season with salt. Mix and close the lid.
4. Place the garlic, tomatillos, onion, serrano peppers, and capers in a parchment-lined baking tray. Season with salt and drizzle with olive oil.
5. Place in the grill and cook for 15 minutes.
6. Remove the vegetables from the grill and transfer to a blender. Add the cilantro and sugar. Add more salt if

needed. Pulse until smooth, then set aside.

7. Pour the mixture into the Dutch oven and add in chicken broth and lime juice.
8. Cook for 3 hours and serve.

NUTRITION:

Calories: 430|Fat: 18.4g| Carb: 7.8g| Protein: 56.4g

8. Grilled Lamb Chops with Rosemary

Prep Time: 10 minutes | Cooking Time: 12 minutes | Temperature: 500F| Servings: 4

Ingredients:

- ½ cup extra virgin olive oil
- ¼ cup coarsely chopped onion
- 2 cloves of garlic, minced
- 2 tbsp. soy sauce
- 2 tbsp. balsamic vinegar
- 1 tbsp. fresh rosemary
- 2 tsp. Dijon mustard
- 1 tsp. Worcestershire sauce
- Salt and pepper to taste
- 4 lamb chops (8 ounces each)

Directions:

1. Heat oil in a saucepan and sauté the onion and garlic until fragrant.
2. In a food processor, add soy sauce, vinegar, rosemary, mustard, Worcestershire sauce, salt, and pepper. Pulse until smooth. Set aside.
3. Preheat the Traeger to 500F for 15 minutes with lid closed.
4. Brush the lamb chops on both sides with the paste. Place on the grill grates and cook for 6 minutes per side or until the lamb chops reach 135F for medium-rare.
5. Serve.

NUTRITION:

Calories: 442|Fat: 38.5g| Carb: 6.1g| Protein: 16.7g

9. Rosemary Lamb with Garlic

Prep Time: 10 minutes | Cooking Time: 10 minutes | Temperature: 300F| Servings: 6

Ingredients:

- 2 pounds of lamb loin or rib chops thick cut
- 4 minced garlic cloves garlic
- 1 tbsp. of fresh chopped rosemary
- 1 and ¼ tsp. of kosher salt
- ½ tsp. of ground black pepper
- Zest of 1 lemon
- ¼ cup of olive oil

Directions:

1. Combine the rosemary with garlic, salt, pepper, lemon zest, and olive oil in a bowl.
2. Pour the prepared marinade over the lamb chops and coat well. Marinate in the refrigerator for 1 hour.
3. Preheat the grill to 300F for 15 minutes.
4. Grill the lamb chops over medium-high for 7 to 10 minutes, or until the internal temperature reads 135F.
5. Rest the chops on a plate covered with aluminum foil for 5 minutes.
6. Serve.

NUTRITION:

Calories: 171.5|Fat: 7.8g| Carb: 0.4g| Protein: 23.2g

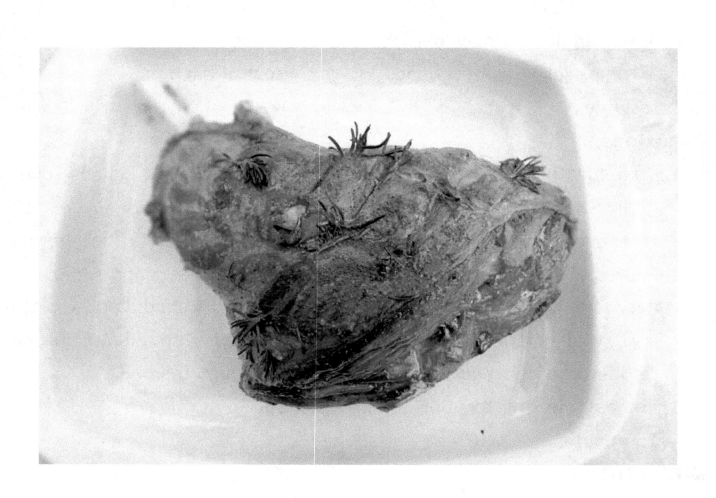

10. Rack of Lamb

Prep Time: 20 minutes | Cooking Time: 75 minutes | Temperature: 200F| Servings: 4

Ingredients:

- 1/2 cup olive oil
- ½ cup dry mustard
- ¼ cup hot chili powder
- 2 tbsp. lemon juice
- 2 tbsp. onion, minced
- 1 tbsp. paprika
- 1 tbsp. dried thyme
- 1 tbsp. salt
- 1 American rack of lamb, 7-9 chops

Mint Sauce

- ¼ cup fresh mint leaves, chopped
- ¼ cup hot water
- 2 tbsp. apple cider vinegar
- 2 tbsp. brown sugar
- ½ tsp. salt
- ½ tsp. fresh ground pepper

Directions:

1. In a small bowl, mix in the olive oil, mustard, chili powder, lemon juice, onion, paprika, thyme, Worcestershire sauce, and salt.
2. Preheat the grill to 200F.
3. Rub the paste all over the lamb and transfer it to the grill. Smoke for 75 minutes or until internal temperature reaches 145F.
4. Remove lamb from the heat and rest for a few minutes.
5. Serve with mint sauce.

NUTRITION:

Calories: 920|Fat: 33g| Carb: 8g| Protein: 52g

11. Mouthwatering Lamb Chops

Prep Time: 15 minutes | Cooking Time: 20 minutes| Temperature: 165F and 450F| Servings: 4

Ingredients:

For Marinade

- o ½ cup of rice wine vinegar
- o 1 tsp. liquid smoke
- o 2 tbsp. extra virgin olive oil
- o 2 tbsp. dried onion, minced
- o 1 tbsp. fresh mint, chopped

Lamb Chops

- o 8 (4 ounces) lamb chops
- o ½ cup hot pepper jelly
- o 1 tbsp. Sriracha
- o 1 tsp. salt
- o 1 tsp. ground black pepper

Directions:

1. In a bowl, whisk in the rice wine vinegar, liquid smoke, olive oil, minced onion, and mint.
2. Add lamb chops in an aluminum roasting pan. Pour marinade over the meat and coat well.
3. Cover with plastic wrap and marinate for 2 hours.
4. Preheat the smoker to 165F.
5. Heat a saucepan over low heat. Add hot pepper jelly and sriracha. Keep it warm.
6. Remove the lamb chops from the marinade and pat dry. Discard marinade.
7. Season chops with salt, pepper, and transfer to the grill grate.
8. Close and smoke for 5 minutes.

9. Remove chops from grill and increase the temperature to 450F.
10. Transfer chops to grill and sear for 2 minutes per side or until internal temperature reaches 145F.
11. Serve.

NUTRITION:

Calories: 227|Fat: 21g| Carb: 0g| Protein: 49g

12. Greek Lamb Leg

Prep Time: 15 minutes | Cooking Time: 25 minutes| Temperature: 325F | Servings: 12

Ingredients:

- 2 tbsp. fresh rosemary, chopped
- 1 tbsp. ground thyme
- 5 garlic cloves, minced
- 2 tbsp. salt
- 1 tbsp. ground pepper
- Butcher's string
- 1 whole boneless (6-8 pounds) leg of lamb
- ¼ cup extra virgin olive oil
- 1 cup red wine vinegar
- ½ cup oil

Directions:

1. In a bowl, add the rosemary, thyme, garlic, salt, pepper, and keep it on the side. Use butcher's string and tie the leg of lamb in the shape of the roast.
2. Rub lamb generously with the olive oil mix and spice mix.
3. Transfer to plate and cover with plastic wrap. Chill for 4 hours
4. Remove lamb from the fridge.
5. Preheat the grill to 325F.
6. In a bowl, add red wine vinegar and oil.
7. Place lamb directly on the grill and close the lid. Smoke 20 to 25 minutes per pound, making sure to keep basting after every 30 minutes.
8. Once the thickest part reaches 145F, the lamb is ready.
9. Rest and serve.

NUTRITION:

Calories: 590|Fat: 50g| Carb: 3g| Protein: 55g

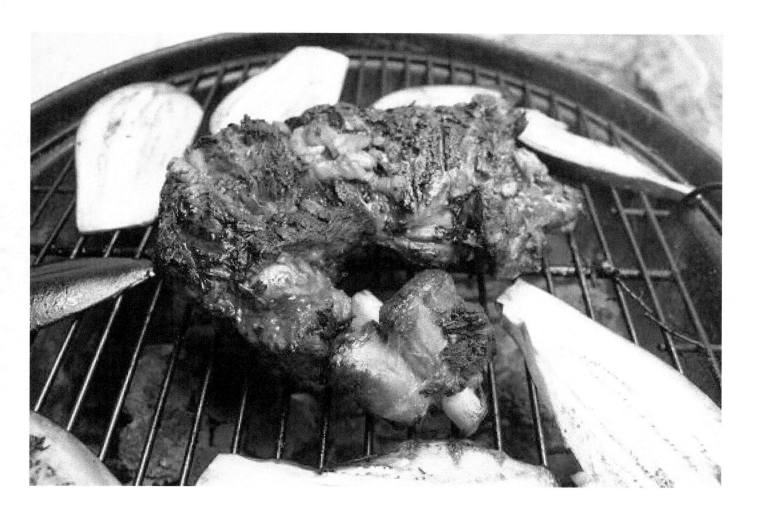

PORK RECIPES

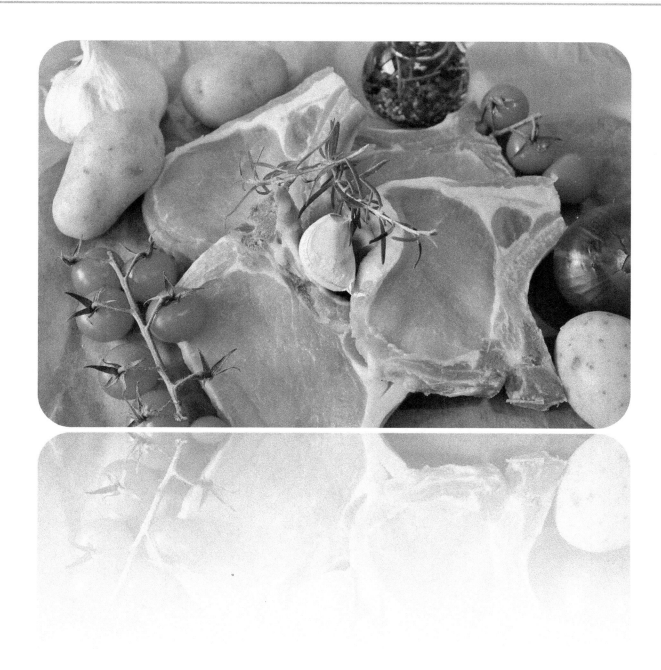

13. Wet-Rubbed St. Louis Ribs

Prep Time: 15 minutes| Cooking Time: 4 hours | Temperature: 180F & 250F| Servings: 3

Ingredients:

- 1/2 cup brown sugar
- 1 tbsp cumin, ground
- 1 tbsp Ancho Chile powder
- 1 tbsp smoked paprika
- 1 tbsp garlic salt
- 3 tbsp balsamic vinegar
- 1 Rack St. Louis style ribs
- 2 cups apple juice

Directions:

1. Add all the ingredients except ribs in a bowl and mix until well mixed. Place the rub on both sides of the ribs and let sit for 10 minutes.
2. Preheat the grill to 180F for 15 minutes. Smoke the ribs for 2 hours.
3. Increase the temperature to 250F and wrap the ribs and apple juice with foil.
4. Place back the pork and cook for 2 hours more.
5. Remove from the grill and rest for 10 minutes. Serve.

NUTRITION:

Calories: 210|Fat: 13g| Carb: 0g| Protein: 24g

14. Cocoa Crusted Pork Tenderloin

Prep Time: 30 minutes | Cooking Time: 25 minutes | Temperature: 400F & 350F | Servings: 5

Ingredients:

- 1 pork tenderloin
- 1/2 tbsp fennel, ground
- 2 tbsp cocoa powder, unsweetened
- 1 tbsp smoked paprika
- 1/2 tbsp kosher salt
- 1/2 tbsp black pepper
- 1 tbsp extra virgin olive oil
- 3 green onion

Directions:

1. Combine everything in a bowl, except for the pork loin.
2. Rub the mixture on the pork and refrigerate for 30 minutes.
3. Preheat the grill to 400F for 15 minutes with lid closed.
4. Sear all sides of the loin at the front of the grill, then reduce the temperature to 350F and move the pork to the center grill.
5. Cook for 15 more minutes or until the internal temperature reaches 145F.
6. Remove from the grill and rest for 10 minutes.
7. Slice and serve.

NUTRITION:

Calories: 264|Fat: 13.1g| Carb: 4.6g| Protein: 33g

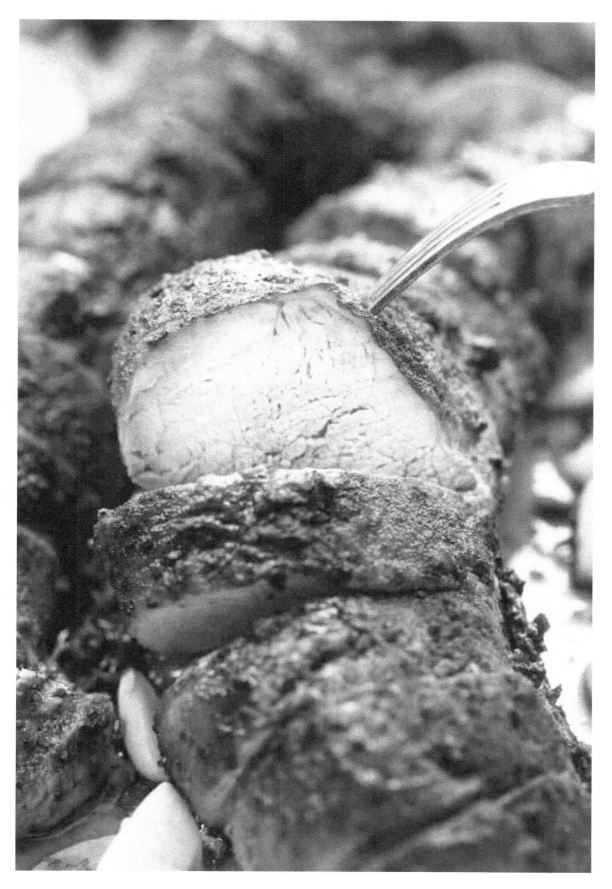

15. Smoked Apple Pork Tenderloin

Prep Time: 10 minutes | Cooking Time: 3 hours | Temperature: 225F|
Servings: 6

Ingredients:

- ½ cup apple juice
- 3 tbsp. honey
- 3 tbsp. Traeger Pork and Poultry Rub
- ¼ cup brown sugar
- 2 tbsp. thyme leaves
- ½ tbsp. black pepper
- 2 pork tenderloin roasts, skin removed

Directions:

1. In a bowl, mix the apple juice, honey, pork, and poultry rub, brown sugar, thyme, and black pepper. Mix well.
2. Add the pork loins into the marinade and allow to soak for 3 hours in the fridge.
3. Preheat the grill to 225F. Close the lid and preheat for 15 minutes.
4. Place the marinated pork loin on the grill grate and cook until the temperature reaches 145F. cook for 2 to 3 hours on low heat.
5. Meanwhile, place the marinade in a saucepan. Place the saucepan in the grill and allow it to simmer until the sauce has reduced.
6. Before taking the meat out, baste the pork with the reduced marinade.
7. Rest and serve.

NUTRITION:

Calories: 203|Fat: 3.6g| Carb: 15.4g| Protein: 26.4g

16. BBQ Pork Ribs

Prep Time: 10 minutes | Cooking Time: 2 hours | Temperature: 225F|
Servings: 6

Ingredients:

- 2 racks of St. Louis-style ribs
- 1 cup Traeger Pork and Poultry Rub
- 1/8 cup brown sugar
- 4 tbsp. butter
- 4 tbsp. agave
- 1 bottle Traeger Sweet and Heat BBQ Sauce

Directions:

1. In a bowl, combine the Traeger Pork and Poultry Rub, brown sugar, butter, and agave. Mix well.
2. Massage the rub onto the ribs and allow them to rest in the fridge for minimum of 2 hours.
3. Fire the Traeger Grill to 225F. Close the lid and preheat for 15 minutes.
4. Place the ribs on the grill grate and close the lid. Smoke for 1 hour and 30 minutes. Flip the ribs halfway through the cooking time.
5. Brush the ribs with the BBQ sauce ten minutes before the cooking time ends.
6. Remove from the grill and allow to rest before slicing.

NUTRITION:

Calories: 399|Fat:20.5g | Carb: 3.5g| Protein: 47.2g

17. Smoked Apple BBQ Ribs

Prep Time: 10 minutes | Cooking Time: 2 hours | Temperature: 225F | Servings: 6

Ingredients:

- 2 racks St. Louis-style ribs
- ¼ cup Traeger Big Game Rub
- 1 cup apple juice
- A bottle of Traeger BBQ Sauce

Directions:

1. In a bowl, mix the game rub and apple juice until mixed well.
2. Massage the run onto the ribs and allow them to rest in the fridge for at least 2 hours.
3. Fire the Traeger Grill to 225F. Close the lid and preheat for 15 minutes.
4. Place the ribs on the grill grate and close the lid. Smoke for 1 hour and 30 minutes. Flip the ribs halfway through the cooking time.
5. Brush the ribs with BBQ sauce, ten minutes before the cooking time ends.
6. Rest and serve.

NUTRITION:

Calories: 337|Fat: 12.9g| Carb: 4.7g| Protein: 47.1g

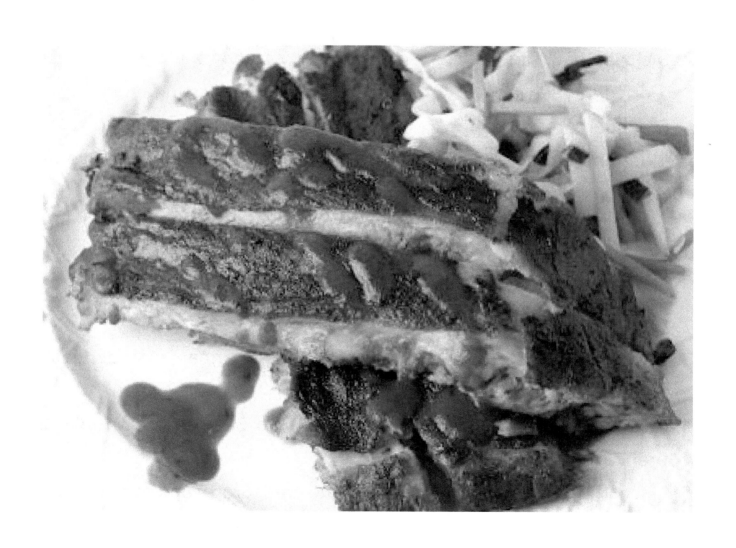

18. Citrus-Brained Pork Roast

Prep Time: 10 minutes | Cooking Time: 45 minutes | Temperature: 300F| Servings: 6

Ingredients:

- ½ cup of salt
- ¼ cup brown sugar
- 3 cloves of garlic, minced
- 2 dried bay leaves
- 6 peppercorns
- 1 lemon, juiced
- ½ tsp. dried fennel seeds
- ½ tsp. red pepper flakes
- ½ cup of apple juice
- ½ cup of orange juice
- 5 pounds pork loin
- 2 tbsp. extra virgin olive oil

Directions:

1. In a bowl, combine the salt, brown sugar, garlic, bay leaves, peppercorns, lemon juice, fennel seeds, pepper flakes, apple juice, and orange juice.
2. Mix to form a paste rub.
3. Rub the mixture onto the pork loin and marinate for at least 2 hours.
4. Add in the oil and fire the Traeger Grill to 300F. Close the lid and preheat for 15 minutes.
5. Place the seasoned pork loin on the grill grate and close the lid. Cook for 45 minutes. Flip the pork halfway through the cooking time.
6. Serve.

NUTRITION:

Calories: 869 |Fat: 43.9g| Carb: 15.2g| Protein: 97.2g

19. Pork Collar and Rosemary Marinade

Prep Time: 15 minutes| Cooking Time: 30 minutes | Temperature: 450F & 325F| Servings: 6

Ingredients:

- 1 pork collar, 3-4 pounds
- 3 tbsp. rosemary, fresh
- 3 shallots, minced
- 2 tbsp. garlic, chopped
- ½ cup bourbon
- 2 tsp. coriander, ground
- 1 bottle of apple ale
- 1 tsp. ground black pepper
- 2 tsp. salt
- 3 tbsp. oil

Directions:

1. In a zip lock bag, add everything except the meat. Mix well.
2. Cut meat into slabs and add them to the marinade. Let it refrigerate overnight.
3. Preheat, the smoker to 450F.
4. Transfer meat to smoker and smoke for 5 minutes. Lower temperature to 325F and pour marinade all over and cook for 25 minutes or until the internal temperature reaches 160F.
5. Serve.

NUTRITION:

Calories: 420|Fat: 26g| Carb: 4g| Protein: 59g

20. Roasted Ham

Prep Time: 15 minutes | Cooking Time: 2 hours 15 minutes | Temperature: 325F| Servings: 6

Ingredients:

- 8-10 pounds ham, bone-in
- 2 tbsp. mustard, Dijon
- ¼ cup horseradish
- 1 bottle BBQ Apricot Sauce

Directions:

1. Preheat, the smoker to 325F.
2. Cover a roasting pan with foil and place the ham, transfer to the smoker, and smoke for 1 hour and 30 minutes.
3. Take a small pan and add sauce, mustard, and horseradish. Place it over medium heat and cook for a few minutes. Keep it on the side.
4. After 1 hour 30 minutes of smoking, glaze ham and smoke for 30 minutes more until the internal temperature reaches 135F.
5. Rest for 20 minutes, slice, and serve.

NUTRITION:

Calories:460 |Fat: 43g| Carb: 10g| Protein: 64g

21. Smoked Pork Loin

Prep Time: 15 minutes | Cooking Time: 3 hours | Temperature: 250F | Servings: 6

Ingredients:

- ½ quart apple juice
- ½ quart apple cider vinegar
- ½ cup of sugar
- ¼ cup of salt
- 2 tbsp. fresh ground pepper
- 1 pork loin roast
- ½ cup Greek seasoning

Directions:

1. Take a large container and make the brine mix by adding apple juice, vinegar, salt, pepper, sugar, liquid smoke, and mix.
2. Keep stirring until the sugar and salt dissolved, and add the loin.
3. Add more water if needed to submerge the meat.
4. Cover and chill overnight.
5. Preheat the grill to 250F.
6. Coat the meat with the Greek seasoning and transfer it to your smoker.
7. Smoke for 3 hours or until the internal temperature of the thickest part reaches 160F.
8. Serve and enjoy.

NUTRITION:

Calories: 169 |Fat: 5g| Carb: 3g | Protein: 77g

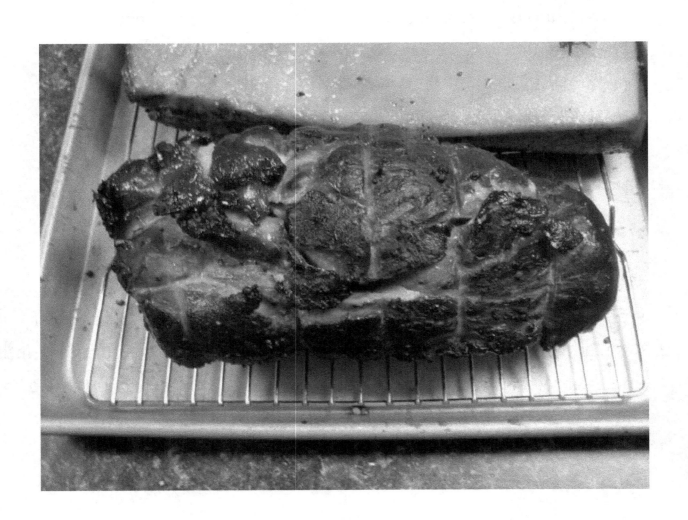

22. Smoke Pulled Pork

Prep Time: 15 minutes | Cooking Time: 3 hours| Temperature: 250F| Servings: 4

Ingredients:

- 6-9 lb. of whole pork shoulder
- 2 cups of apple cider
- Big game rub

Directions:

1. Set the temperature to 250F and preheat by keeping the lid closed for 15 minutes.
2. Season the pork with a big game rub on all sides.
3. Put the pork on the grill grate, keep the fat side up.
4. Smoke for 3 to 5 hours or until the internal temperature reaches 160F.
5. Remove it from the grill and keep it aside.
6. Now take a baking sheet and keep 4 large pieces of aluminum foil, one on top of the other. This should be enough to wrap the pork entirely.
7. Keep the pork in the very center of the oil and bring up the side a little. Pour apple cider on top of the pork and wrap the foil tightly around it.
8. Keep it back on the grill again, having the fat side up, and cook till the internal temperature reaches 200F. This should take 3 to 4 hours.
9. Remove it from the grill and let it rest for 45 minutes inside the foil packet.
10. Take off the foil and pour off the extra liquid.

11. Now keep the pork in a dish and remove the bones and excess fat.
12. Add the separated liquid back to the pork and season it again with a big game rub.
13. Serve.

NUTRITION:

Calories: 196|Fat: 5g| Carb: 3g| Protein: 44g

23. Easy Pork Chunk Roast

Prep Time: 15 minutes | Cooking Time: 4 hours | Temperature: 225F|
Servings: 6

Ingredients:

- 1 whole 4-5 pounds chuck roast
- ¼ cup olive oil
- ¼ cup firm packed brown sugar
- 2 tbsp. Cajun seasoning
- 2 tbsp. paprika
- 2 tbsp. cayenne pepper

Directions:

1. Preheat the grill to 225F.
2. Rub chuck roast all over with olive oil.
3. In a small bowl, add the brown sugar, paprika, Cajun seasoning, cayenne, and mix.
4. Coat the roast well with the spice mix.
5. Transfer the chuck roast to the grill rack and smoke for 4 to 5 hours, or until the internal temperature reaches 165F.
6. Rest and enjoy.

NUTRITION:

Calories: 219|Fat: 16g| Carb: 0g| Protein: 59g

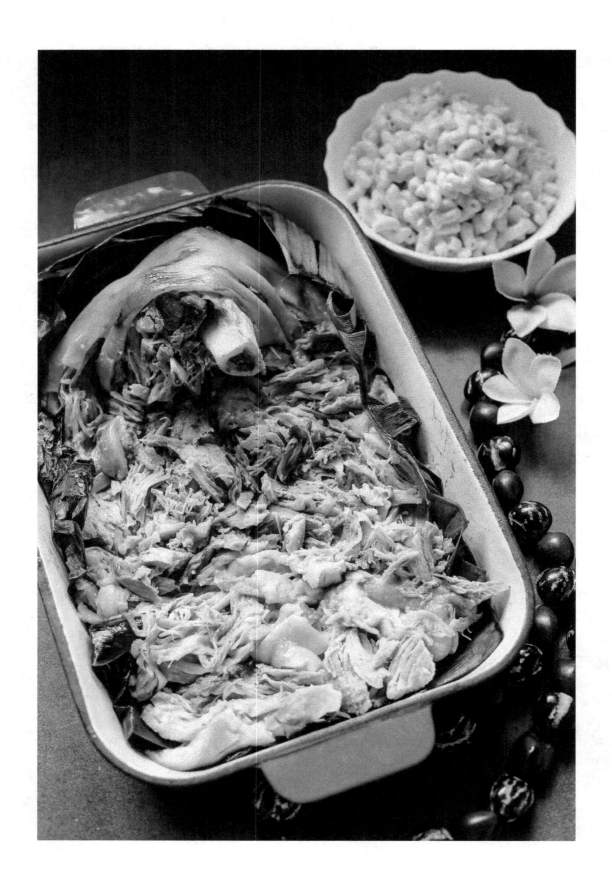

24. Pineapple Pork BBQ

Prep Time: 10 minutes | Cooking Time: 1 hour | Temperature: 300F|
Servings: 4

Ingredients:

- 1-pound pork sirloin
- 4 cups pineapple juice
- 3 cloves garlic, minced
- 1 cup carne asada marinade
- 2 tbsp. salt
- 1 tsp. ground black pepper

Directions:

1. Place everything except for the pork in a bowl and mix well.
2. Massage the pork with this mixture. Place inside the fridge to marinate for at least 2 hours.
3. Fire the Traeger to 300F. Close the lid and preheat for 15 minutes.
4. Place the pork sirloin on the grill grate and cook for 45 to 60 minutes. Flip once at the halfway mark.
5. Meanwhile, place the marinade in a pan and place it inside the smoker. Allow the marinade to cook and reduce.
6. Baste the pork sirloin with the reduced marinade before cooking time ends.
7. Serve.

NUTRITION:

Calories: 347|Fat: 23g| Carb: 12g| Protein: 53.4g

25. BBQ Spareribs with Mandarin Glaze

Prep Time: 10 minutes | Cooking Time: 60 minutes | Temperature: |
Servings: 6

Ingredients:

- 3 large spareribs, membrane removed
- 3 tbsp. yellow mustard
- 1 tbsp. Worcestershire sauce
- 1 cup honey
- 1 ½ cup brown sugar
- 13 ounces Traeger Mandarin Glaze
- 1 tsp. sesame oil
- 1 tsp. soy sauce
- 1 tsp. garlic powder

Directions:

1. In a bowl, mix everything except for the meat.
2. Massage the spice mixture onto the spareribs. Rest in the fridge for at least 3 hours.
3. Fire the Traeger to 300F. Close the lid and preheat for 15 minutes.
4. Place the seasoned ribs on the grill grate and cover the lid.
5. Cook for 60 minutes.
6. Rest. Slice and serve.

NUTRITION:

Calories: 123|Fat:36.9g | Carb: 10.3g| Protein: 76.8g

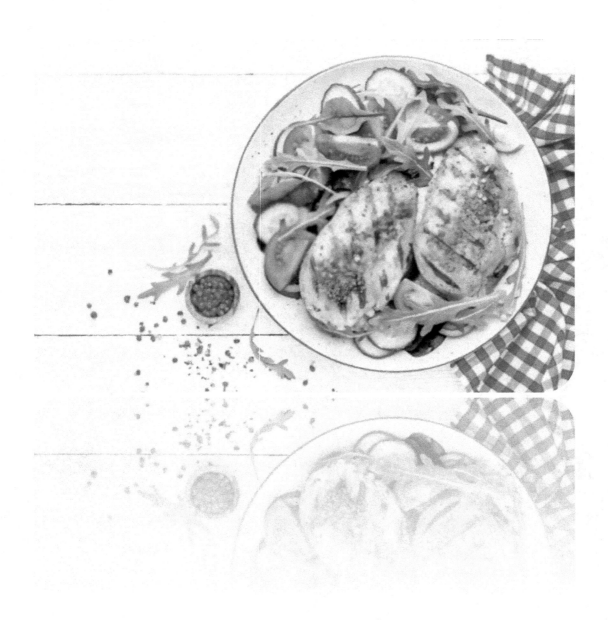

26. Lemon Chicken Breast

Prep Time: 15 min| Cooking Time: 30 minutes | Temperature: 400F | Servings: 4

Ingredients:

- 6 chicken breasts, skinless and boneless
- ½ cup oil
- 1-3 fresh thyme sprigs
- 1 teaspoon ground black pepper
- 2 teaspoon salt
- 2 teaspoons honey
- 1 garlic clove, chopped
- 1 lemon, juiced, and zested
- Lemon wedges

Directions:

1. In a bowl, prepare the marinade by mixing lemon zest, juice, garlic, honey, salt, pepper, and thyme. Add oil and whisk.
2. Place the chicken in a Ziplock bag along with the marinade and let them sit in the fridge for 4 hours.
3. Preheat, the smoker to 400F
4. Drain chicken and smoke until the chicken reaches 165F, about 15 minutes.
5. Serve.

NUTRITION:

Calories: 230 |Fat: 7g| Carb: 1g| Protein: 38g

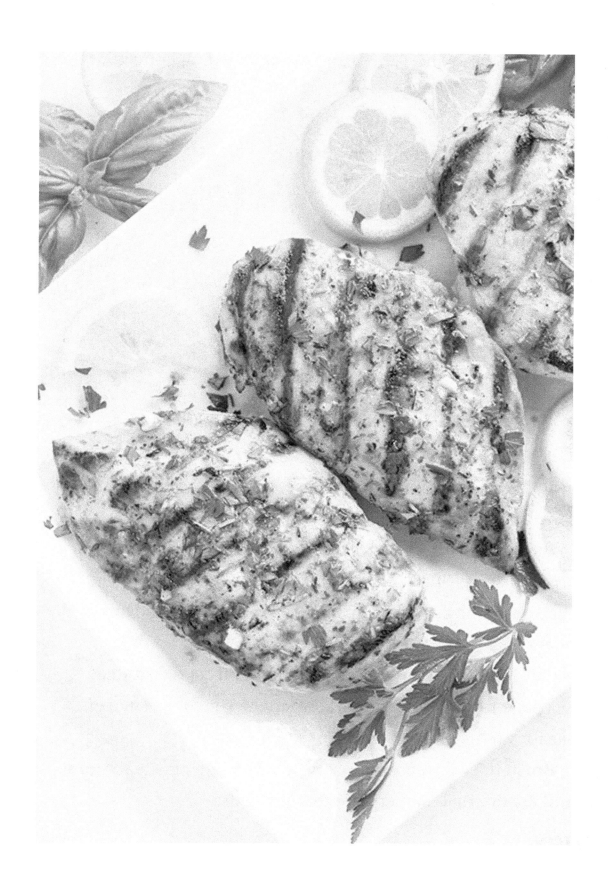

27. Maple and Bacon Chicken

Prep Time: 20 min| Cooking Time: 1 and ½ hours | Temperature: 250F |Servings: 7

Ingredients:

- o   4 boneless and skinless chicken breasts
- o   Salt as needed
- o   Fresh pepper
- o   12 slices bacon, uncooked
- o   1 cup maple syrup
- o   ½ cup melted butter
- o   1 teaspoon liquid smoke

Directions:

1. Preheat, the smoker to 250F.
2. Season chicken with salt and pepper.
3. Wrap the breast with 3 bacon slices and cover the entire surface.
4. Secure the bacon with toothpicks.
5. In a bowl, add the maple syrup, butter, liquid smoke, and mix well.
6. Reserve 1/3 of the mixture for later use.
7. Submerge the chicken breast into the butter mix and coat well.
8. Place a pan on your smoker and transfer chicken to the smoker.
9. Smoke for 1 to 1 ½ hour.
10.   Brush the chicken with reserved butter and smoke for 30 minutes more or until the internal temperature reaches 165F.

NUTRITION:

Calories: 458|Fat: 20g| Carb: 5g| Protein: 65g

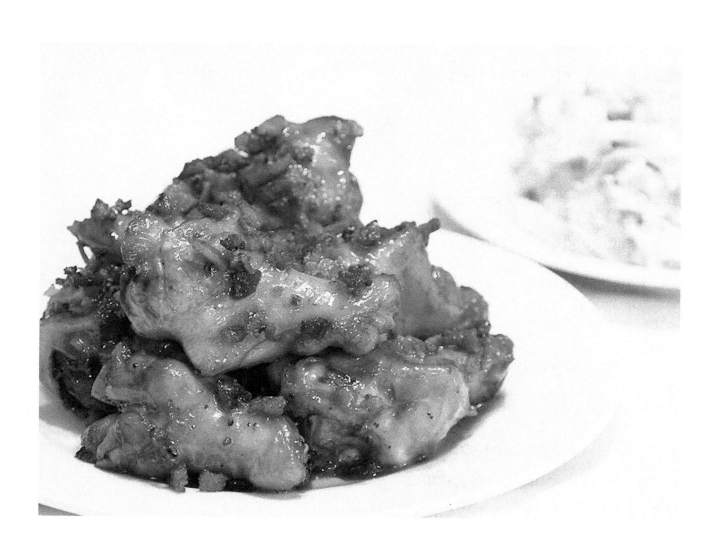

28. Paprika Chicken

Prep Time: 20 minutes | Cooking Time: 2 hours | Temperature: 220F | Servings: 7

Ingredients:

- o 6 chicken breasts
- o 4 tablespoons olive oil
- o 2 tablespoons smoked paprika
- o ½ tablespoon salt
- o ¼ teaspoon pepper
- o 2 teaspoons garlic powder
- o 2 teaspoons garlic salt
- o 2 teaspoons pepper
- o 1 teaspoon cayenne pepper
- o 1 teaspoon rosemary

Directions:

1. Preheat, the smoker to 220F.
2. Prepare the chicken breast and transfer it to a greased baking dish.
3. In a bowl, add the spices and mix well.
4. Press the spice mix over the chicken and transfer it to the chicken to the smoker.
5. Smoke for 1 and ½ hours.
6. Turn over and cook for 30 minutes more, or until the internal temperature reaches 165F.
7. Cover with foil and allow to rest for 15 minutes. Serve.

NUTRITION:

Calories: 237|Fat: 6.1g| Carb: 14g| Protein: 38g

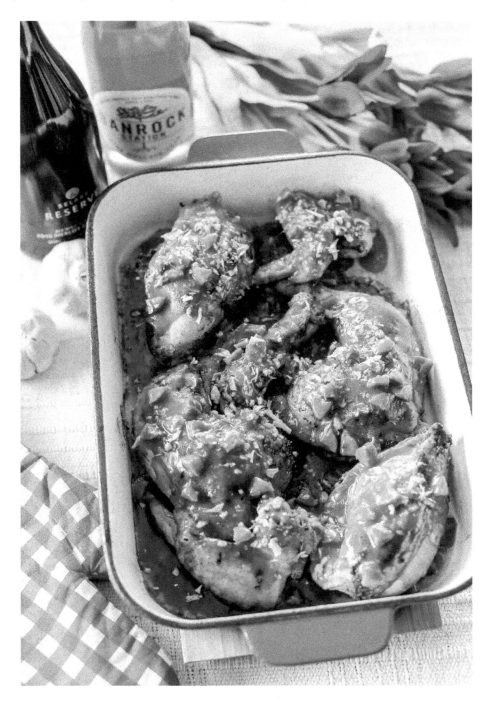

29. Sweet Sriracha BBQ Chicken

Prep Time: 30 minutes | Cooking Time: 1-hour ½ hours to 2 hours | Temperature: 250F | Servings: 5

Ingredients:

o   1 cup sriracha

o   ½ cup butter

o   ½ cup molasses

o   ½ cup ketchup

o   ¼ cup firmly packed brown sugar

o   1 teaspoon salt

o   1 teaspoon fresh ground black pepper

o   1 whole chicken, cut into pieces

o   ½ teaspoon fresh parsley leaves, chopped

Directions:

1. Preheat, the smoker to 250F.
2. In a pan, add salt, pepper, mustard, brown sugar, molasses, ketchup, sriracha, and butter. Mix until sugar dissolves.
3. Divide the sauce into two portions.
4. Brush the chicken with half of the sauce and reserve the remaining for service.
5. Transfer chicken to your smoker and smoke for 1 ½ hour to 2 hours or until chicken reaches 165F.
6. Sprinkle the chicken with parsley and serve with sauce.

NUTRITION:

Calories: 148|Fat: 0.6g| Carb: 10g| Protein: 35g

30. Smoked Chicken Drumsticks

Prep Time: 10 min| Cooking Time: 2 hours 30 min| Temperature: 250F | Servings: 5

Ingredients:

- o 10 chicken drumsticks
- o 2 tsp garlic powder
- o 1 tsp salt
- o 1 tsp onion powder
- o 1/2 tsp ground black pepper
- o ½ tsp cayenne pepper
- o 1 tsp brown sugar
- o 1/3 cup hot sauce
- o 1 tsp paprika
- o ½ tsp thyme

Directions:

1. In a bowl, combine salt, pepper, cayenne, thyme, paprika, hot sauce, sugar, and garlic powder. Add the drumsticks and mix.
2. Cover the bowl and refrigerate for 1 hour.
3. Remove the drumsticks from the marinade and let them sit for 1 hour to come to room temperature.
4. Arrange the drumsticks into a rack.
5. Preheat the grill to 250F.
6. Smoke for 2 hours 30 minutes or until drumsticks reaches 180F.
7. Serve.

NUTRITION:

Calories: 167|Fat: 5.4g| Carb: 2.6g| Protein: 25.7g

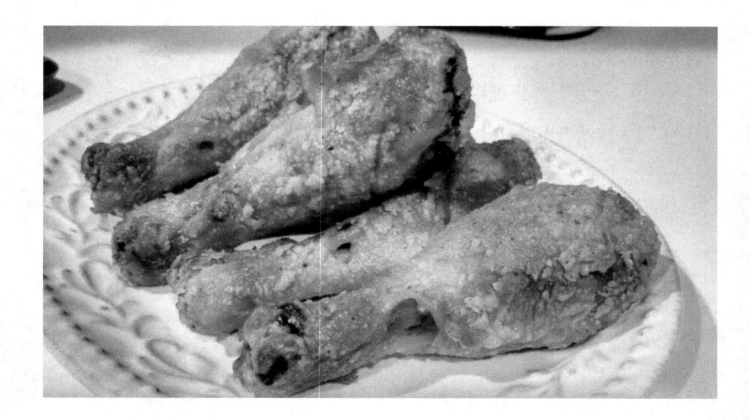

31. Smoked Whole Duck

Prep Time: 15 minutes | Cooking Time: 2 hours 30 minutes | Temperature: 325F | Servings: 6

Ingredients:

- 5 pounds whole duck (trimmed of any excess fat) giblets removed
- 1 small onion (quartered)
- 1 apple (wedged)
- 1 orange (quartered)
- 1 tbsp freshly chopped parsley
- 1 tbsp freshly chopped sage
- ½ tsp onion powder
- 2 tsp smoked paprika
- 1 tsp dried Italian seasoning
- 1 tbsp dried Greek seasoning
- 1 tsp pepper or to taste
- 1 tsp sea salt or to taste

Directions:

1. Rinse duck and pat dry.
2. Use a sharp knife to cut the duck skin all over. Do not cut through the meat. Tie the duck legs together with butcher's string.
3. Combine the Italian seasoning, green seasonings, paprika, salt, pepper, and onion powder to make a rub.

4. Insert the onion, orange, and apple into the duck cavity. Stuff duck with chopped parsley and sage.
5. Season all sides of the duck with rub mixture.
6. Preheat the grill to 325F for 10 minutes.
7. Place duck on the grill grate and roast for 2 to 2 ½ hours, or until the duck reaches 160F.
8. Remove from heat and rest for a few minutes. Cut and serve.

NUTRITION:

Calories: 809 |Fat: 42.9g| Carb: 11.7g| Protein: 89.6g

32. Chicken Fajitas

Prep Time: 5 min | Cooking Time: 20 minutes | Temperature: 450F | Servings: 10

Ingredients:

- 2 lbs., chicken breast, thin sliced

- 1 large red bell pepper

- 1 large onion

- 1 large orange bell pepper

Seasoning mix

- 2 tbsp oil

- ½ tbsp onion powder

- ½ tbsp granulated garlic

- 1 tbsp salt

Directions:

1. Preheat the grill to 450F.
2. Mix seasonings and oil.
3. Add the chicken slices to the mix.
4. Heat a lined pan for 10 minutes.
5. Place the peppers, chicken, and other vegetables in the grill and grill for 10 minutes or until the chicken is cooked.
6. Serve.

NUTRITION:

Calories: 225|Fat: 6g| Carb: 5g| Protein: 29g

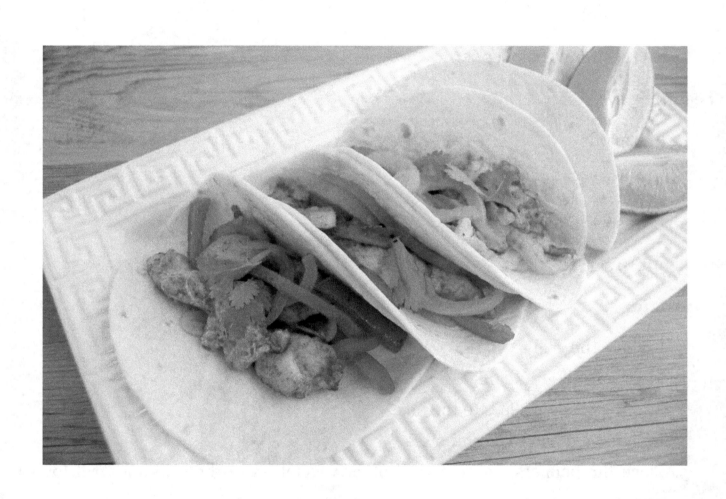

33. Smoked Cornish Chicken

Prep Time: 0 min | Cooking Time: 1 hour 10 minutes | Temperature: 275F & 400F| Servings: 6

Ingredients:

- o   6 Cornish hens

- o   3 tbsp. avocado oil

- o   6 tbsp. spice mix

Directions:

1. Preheat the grill to 275F.
2. Rub the whole hen with oil and spice mix.
3. Place the hen on the grill, breast side down, and smoke for 30 minutes.
4. Flip and increase the temperature to 400F.
5. Cook until the hen reaches 165F.
6. Remove, rest, and serve.

NUTRITION:

Calories: 220 |Fat: 18g| Carb: 1g| Protein: 57g

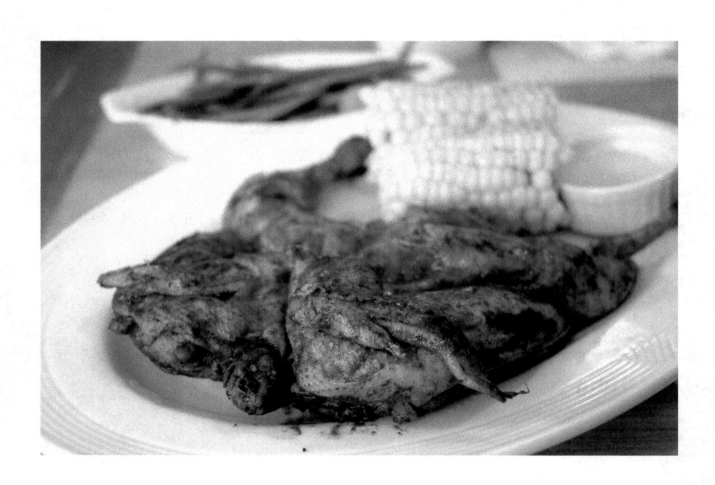

34. Turkey Egg Rolls

Prep Time: 10 minu | Cooking Time: 40 minutes | Temperature: 350F | Servings: 4

Ingredients:

- ½ cup corn
- 2 cups leftover wild turkey meat
- ½ cup black beans
- 3 tbsp. Taco seasoning
- ½ cup water
- 1 can Rotel chilies and tomatoes
- 12 egg roll wrappers
- 4 cloves of minced garlic
- 1 chopped Poblano pepper
- ½ cup chopped white onion

Directions:

1. Heat olive oil in a skillet.
2. Add onions and peppers and cook for 3 minutes.
3. Add garlic and cook for 30 seconds more. Add chilies and beans to the mixture. Reduce the heat and simmer for 5 minutes.
4. Add the taco seasoning, meat and cook for 5 minutes. Add ½ cup water and cook until everything is heated all the way through.
5. Remove the content from the heat and box it to store in a refrigerator.
6. Place a spoonful of the cooked mixture in each wrapper and then wrap it tightly. Repeat.

7. Preheat the grill to 350F and brush with some oil. Cook the egg rolls for 15 minutes or until both sides are crispy.
8. Serve.

NUTRITION:

Calories: 325|Fat: 4.2g| Carb: 26.1g| Protein: 9.2g

35. Hellfire Chicken Wings

Prep Time: 15 min | Cooking Time: 40 minutes | Temperature: 350F | Servings: 6

Ingredients:

- o 3 pounds chicken wings, tips removed
- o 2 tablespoons olive oil

For the Rub:

- o 1 teaspoon onion powder
- o 1 teaspoon salt
- o 1 teaspoon garlic powder
- o 1 tablespoon paprika
- o 1 teaspoon ground black pepper
- o 1 teaspoon celery seed
- o 1 teaspoon cayenne pepper
- o 2 teaspoons brown sugar

For the Sauce:

- o 4 jalapeno peppers, sliced crosswise
- o 8 tablespoons butter, unsalted
- o 1/2 cup hot sauce
- o 1/2 cup cilantro leaves

Directions:

1. Preheat the grill to 350F for 15 minutes.

2. Cut each chicken wing through the joint into two pieces.

3. Place all the rub ingredients in a bowl and mix well. Rub the chicken with this mixture.

4. Place the chicken wings on the grill gate and smoke for 40 minutes or until golden brown. Turning halfway.

5. Meanwhile, prepare the sauce. In a pan, melt the butter, add jalapeno, and cook for 4 minutes.

6. Then stir in hot sauce and cilantro until mix well. Remove the pan from the heat.

7. When done, transfer chicken wings to a dish, top with prepared sauce. Mix and serve.

NUTRITION:

Calories: 250 |Fat: 15g| Carb: 11g| Protein: 19g

36. Spicy BBQ Chicken

Prep Time: 8 hours and 10 minutes | Cooking Time: 3 hours | Temperature: 300F | Servings: 6

Ingredients:

- o   1 whole chicken, cleaned

For the Marinade:

- o   1 medium white onion, peeled

- o   6 Thai chilies

- o   5 cloves of garlic, peeled

- o   1 scotch bonnet

- o   3 tablespoons salt

- o   2 tablespoons sugar

- o   2 tablespoons sweet paprika

- o   4 cups grapeseed oil

Directions:

1. In a food processor, pulse all the marinade ingredients and process until smooth.
2. Rub the chicken with marinade and let it marinate in the refrigerator for 8 hours.
3. Preheat the grill to 300F for 15 minutes.
4. Place the chicken on the grill grate (breast-side up). Smoke for 3 hours or until the chicken reaches 165F.
5. Remove from heat and rest for 15 minutes. Slice and serve.

NUTRITION:

Calories: 190 |Fat: 2.8g| Carb: 8| Protein: 35g

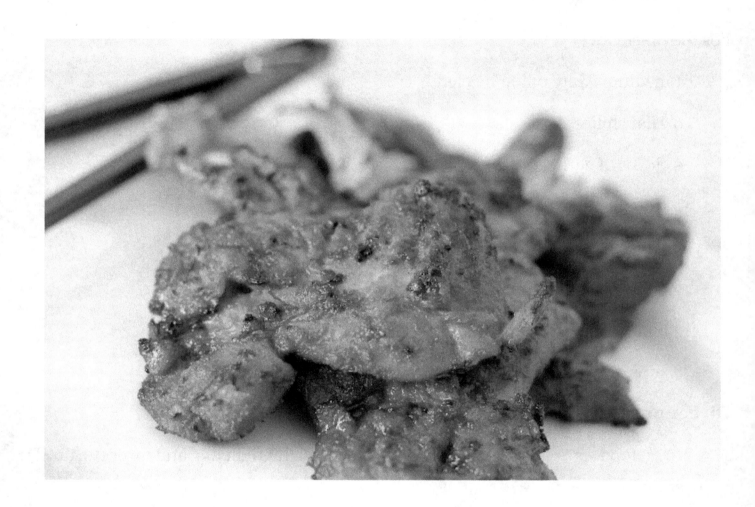

37. Chicken Lollipops

Prep Time: 30 minutes | Cooking Time: 2 hours| Temperature: 300F|
Servings: 6

Ingredients:

- 12 chicken lollipops
- Chicken seasoning
- 10 tbsp. butter, sliced into 12 cubes
- 1 cup barbecue sauce
- 1 cup hot sauce

Directions:

1. Preheat the grill to 300F.
2. Season the chicken with chicken seasoning.
3. Arrange chicken in a baking pan.
4. Put the butter cubes on top of each chicken.
5. Cook the chicken lollipops for 2 hours, basting with the melted butter in the baking pan every 20 minutes.
6. Pour in the barbecue sauce and hot sauce over the chicken.
7. Grill for 15 minutes. Serve.

NUTRITION:

Calories: 935|Fat: 53g| Carb: 4g| Protein: 107g

38. Holiday Turkey Breast

Prep Time: 15 minutes | Cooking Time: 4 hours| Temperature: 250F|
Servings: 6

Ingredients:

- ½ cup honey
- ¼ cup dry sherry
- 1 tbsp. butter
- 2 tbsp. fresh lemon juice
- Salt, to taste
- 1 (3-3½-pound) skinless, boneless turkey breast

Directions:

1. In a pan, place honey, sherry, and butter over low heat and cook until the mixture becomes smooth, stirring continuously.
2. Remove from the heat and stir in the lemon juice and salt. Set aside to cool.
3. Transfer the honey mixture and turkey breast to a sealable bag.
4. Seal the bag and shake to coat well.
5. Refrigerate for 6 to 10 hours.
6. Set the temperature of Traeger to 250F and preheat with a closed lid for 15 minutes.
7. Place the turkey breast onto the grill and cook for 2 ½ to 4 hours or until the desired doneness.
8. Remove turkey breast from grill rest for 20 minutes'.
9. Cut and serve.

NUTRITION:

Calories: 443|Fat: 11.4g| Carb:23.7g | Protein: 59.2g

39. Chinese Inspired Duck Legs

Prep Time: 15 minutes | Cooking Time: 10 minutes | Temperature: 235F| Servings: 8

Ingredients:

For Glaze:

- ¼ cup fresh orange juice
- ¼ cup orange marmalade
- ¼ cup mirin
- 2 tbsp. hoisin sauce
- ½ tsp. red pepper flakes, crushed

For Duck:

- 1 tsp. kosher salt
- ¾ tsp. ground black pepper
- ¾ tsp. Chinese five-spice powder
- 8 (6-oz.) duck legs

Directions:

1. Set the temperature of Traeger to 235F and preheat with a closed lid for 15 minutes.
2. For the glaze: In a pan, add all ingredients over medium heat and bring to a gentle boil. Stirring continuously.
3. Remove from heat and set aside.
4. For the rub: in a bowl, mix together salt, black pepper, and five-spice powder.
5. Rub the duck legs with spice rub evenly.
6. Place the duck legs onto the grill, skin side up, and cook for 50 minutes.
7. Coat the duck legs with glaze and cook for 20 minutes, flipping and coating with glaze after every 5 minutes.
8. Serve.

NUTRITION:

Calories: 303|Fat: 10.2g| Carb: 0.1g | Protein: 49.5g

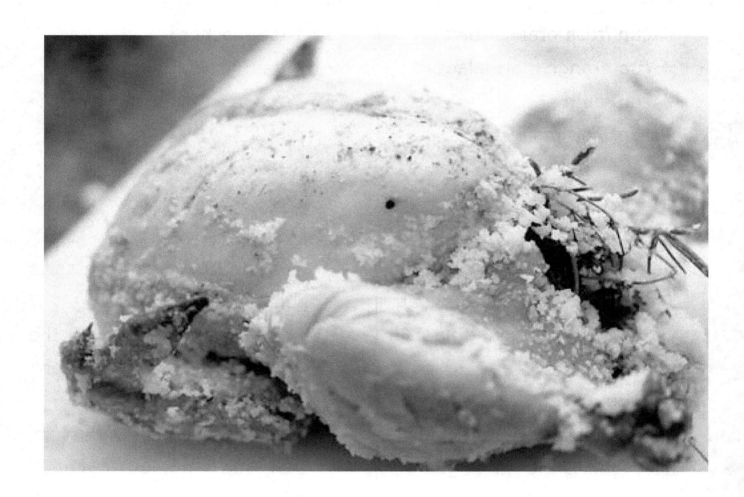

40. Succulent Duck Breast

Prep Time: 10 minutes | Cooking Time: 10 minutes| Temperature: 275F & 400F| Servings: 4

Ingredients:

- 4 (6-oz.) boneless duck breasts
- 2 tbsp. chicken rub

Directions:

1. Set the temperature to Traeger to 275F and preheat with a closed lid for 15 minutes.
2. Score the skin of the duck (with a sharp knife) into a ¼-inch diamond pattern. Season the duck breast with the rub.
3. Place the duck breasts onto the grill, meat side down, and cook for 10 minutes.
4. Now, set the temperature to 400F.
5. Arrange the breasts, skin side down, and cook for 10 minutes, flipping once halfway through.
6. Serve.

NUTRITION:

Calories: 231|Fat: 6.8g| Carb: 1.5g| Protein: 37.4g

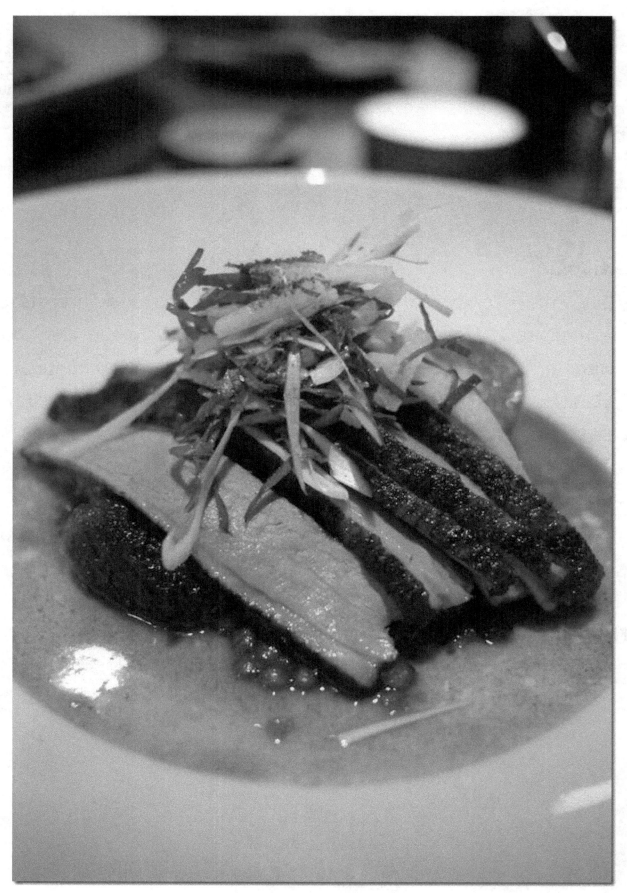

41. Christmas Dinner Goose

Prep Time: 20 minutes| Cooking Time: 3 hours| Temperature: 350F| Servings: 12

Ingredients:

- 1½ cup kosher salt
- 1 cup brown sugar
- 20 cups water
- 1 (12-lb.) whole goose, giblets removed
- 1 navel orange, cut into 6 wedges
- 1 large onion, cut into 8 wedges
- 2 bay leaves
- ¼ cup juniper berries, crushed
- 12 black peppercorns
- Salt and freshly ground black pepper, to taste
- 1 apple, cut into 6 wedges
- 2-3 fresh parsley sprigs

Directions:

1. Trim off any loose neck skin.
2. Then, trim the first two joints off the wings.
3. Wash the goose under cold running water and pat dry with paper towels.
4. With the tip of a paring knife, prick the goose all over the skin.
5. In a pitcher, dissolve salt and brown sugar in water.
6. Squeeze 3 orange wedges into the brine.
7. Add goose, 4 onion wedges, bay leaves, juniper berries, and peppercorns in brine and refrigerate for 24 hours.
8. Set the temperature of Traeger to 350F and preheat with a closed lid for 15 minutes.

9. Remove the goose from brine and pat dry completely.

10. Season the in and outside of goose with salt and black pepper evenly.

11. Stuff the cavity with apple wedges, herbs, remaining orange, and onion wedges.

12. With kitchen strings, tie the legs together loosely.

13. Place the goose onto a rack arranged in a shallow roasting pan.

14. Arrange the goose on the grill and cook for 1 hour.

15. With a basting bulb, remove some of the fat from the pan and cook for 1 hour.

16. Again, remove excess fat from the pan and cook for ½ to 1 hour more.

17. Remove goose from the grill and rest for 20 minutes.

NUTRITION:

Calories: 907|Fat: 36.3g| Carb: 23.5g| Protein: 50.6g

42. Grilled Chicken Kabobs

Prep Time: 45 minutes | Cooking Time: 12 minutes | Temperature: 450F| Servings: 6

Ingredients:

- 1/2 cup olive oil
- 2 tbsp white vinegar
- 1 tbsp lemon juice
- 1-1/2 tbsp salt
- 1/2 tbsp pepper, coarsely ground
- 2 tbsp chives, freshly chopped
- 1-1/2 tbsp thyme, freshly chopped
- 2 tbsp Italian parsley freshly chopped
- 1 tbsp garlic, minced

Kabobs

- 1 each orange, red, and yellow pepper
- 1-1/2 lb. chicken breast, boneless and skinless
- 12 crimini mushrooms

Directions:

1. In a bowl, add all the marinade ingredients and mix well.
2. Toss the chicken and mushrooms in the marinade, then refrigerate for 30 minutes.
3. Meanwhile, soak the skewers in hot water. Remove the chicken from the fridge and assembling the kabobs.
4. Preheat the grill to 450F.
5. Grill the kabobs for 6 minutes. Then flip and grill for 6 minutes more.
6. Remove from the grill and rest. Serve.

NUTRITION:

Calories: 165|Fat: 13g| Carb: 1g| Protein: 33g

43. Grilled Chicken

Prep Time: 10 minutes | Cooking Time: 1 hour 10 minutes|
Temperature: 450F| Servings: 6

Ingredients:

- 5 lb. whole chicken
- 1/2 cup oil
- Chicken rub

Directions:

1. Preheat the grill on smoke with the lid open for 5 minutes.
2. Then close the lid, increase the temperature to 450F and preheat for 15 minutes more.
3. Tie the chicken legs together with the baker's twine, then rub the chicken with oil and coat with chicken rub.
4. Place the chicken on the grill with the breast side up.
5. Grill the chicken for 70 minutes without opening it or until the internal temperature reaches 165F.
6. Remove the chicken and cool for 15 minutes.
7. Serve.

NUTRITION:

Calories: 935|Fat: 53g| Carb: 0g | Protein: 107g

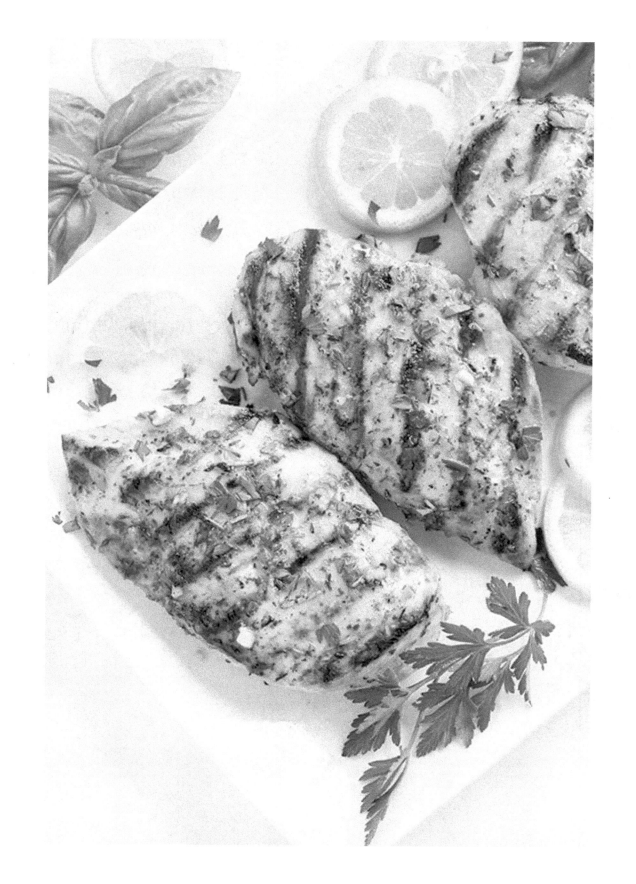

44. Chicken Breasts

Prep Time: 10 minutes | Cooking Time: 15 minutes | Temperature: 375F| Servings: 6

Ingredients:

- 3 chicken breasts
- 1 tbsp avocado oil
- 1/4 tbsp garlic powder

- 1/4 tbsp onion powder
- 3/4 tbsp salt
- 1/4 tbsp pepper

Directions:

1. Preheat the grill to 375F.
2. Half the chicken breasts lengthwise, then coat with avocado oil.
3. Season with onion powder, garlic powder, salt, and pepper on all sides.
4. Place the chicken on the grill and cook for 7 minutes on each side or until the internal temperature reaches 165F.
5. Serve.

NUTRITION:

Calories: 120|Fat: 4g| Carb: 0g| Protein: 19g

45. Smoked Spatchcock Turkey

Prep Time: 30 minutes | Cooking Time: 1 hour 45 minutes | Temperature: 400F & 325F| Servings: 6

Ingredients:

- 1 whole turkey
- 1/2 cup oil
- 1/4 cup chicken rub
- 1 tbsp onion powder
- 1 tbsp garlic powder
- 1 tbsp rubbed sage

Directions:

1. Preheat the grill to 400F.
2. Meanwhile, place the turkey on a platter with the breast side down, then cut on either side of the backbone to remove the spine.
3. Flip the turkey and season on both sides, then place it on the preheated grill or on a pan if you want to catch the drippings.
4. Grill on high for 30 minutes. Then reduce the temperature to 325F and grill for 45 minutes more or until the internal temperature reaches 165F.
5. Remove from the grill and rest for 20 minutes.
6. Slice and serve.

NUTRITION:

Calories: 156|Fat: 16g| Carb: 1g| Protein: 22g

46. Smoked Cornish Hens

Prep Time: 10 minutes | Cooking Time: 1 hour | Temperature: 275F & 400F| Servings: 6

Ingredients:

- 6 Cornish hens
- 3 tbsp. avocado oil
- 6 tbsp. rub of choice

Directions:

1. Preheat the grill to 275F.
2. Rub the hens with the oil and then coat with the rub. Place the hens on the grill with the breast side down.
3. Smoke for 30 minutes. Flip the hens and increase the grill temperature to 400F.
4. Cook until the internal temperature reaches 165F.
5. Remove from the grill and rest for 10 minutes.
6. Serve.

NUTRITION:

Calories: 696|Fat: 50g| Carb: 1g| Protein:57g

47. Smoked and Fried Chicken Wings

Prep Time: 10 minutes | Cooking Time: 2 hours | Temperature: 180F|

Servings: 6

Ingredients:

- 3 lb. chicken wings
- 1 tbsp adobo all-purpose seasoning
- Sauce of your choice

Directions:

1. Preheat the grill to 180F.
2. Meanwhile, coat the chicken wings with seasoning.
3. Place the chicken on the grill and smoke for 2 hours. Flip once.
4. Remove the wings from the grill.
5. Preheat oil to 375F in a frying pan. Drop the wings in batches and fry for 5 minutes or until the skin is crispy.
6. Remove from oil and drain.
7. Serve with sauce.

NUTRITION:

Calories: 755|Fat: 55g| Carb: 24g| Protein: 39g

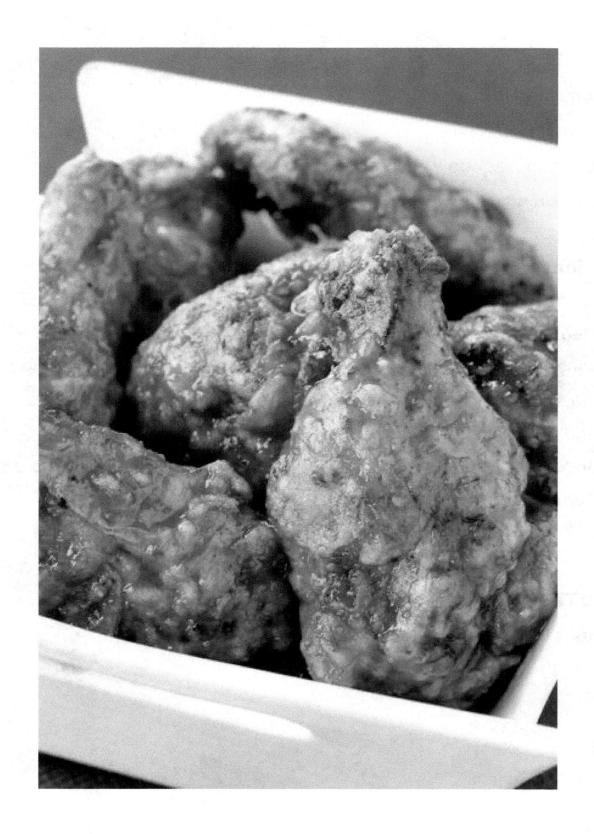

48. Grilled Buffalo Chicken Leg

Prep Time: 5 minutes | Cooking Time: 25 minutes | Temperature: 325F|
Servings: 6

Ingredients:

- 12 chicken legs
- 1/2 tbsp salt
- 1 tbsp buffalo seasoning
- 1 cup buffalo sauce

Directions:

1. Preheat the grill to 325F.
2. Toss the legs in salt and buffalo seasoning, then place them on the preheated grill.
3. Grill for 40 minutes, turn twice.
4. Brush the legs with buffalo sauce and cook for 10 minutes more or until the internal temperature reaches 165F.
5. Remove the legs from the grill, brush with more sauce, and serve.

NUTRITION:

Calories: 956|Fat: 47g| Carb: 1g| Protein: 124g

49. Chili Lime Chicken

Prep Time: 2 minutes | Cooking Time: 15 minutes | Temperature: 400F|
Servings: 1

Ingredients:

- o 1 chicken breast
- o 1 tbsp oil
- o 1 tbsp chile-lime seasoning

Directions:

1. Preheat the grill to 400F.
2. Brush the chicken breast with oil on all sides.
3. Sprinkle with seasoning and salt to taste.
4. Grill for 7 minutes per side or until the internal temperature reaches 165F.
5. Serve.

NUTRITION:

Calories: 131|Fat: 5g| Carb: 4g | Protein: 19g

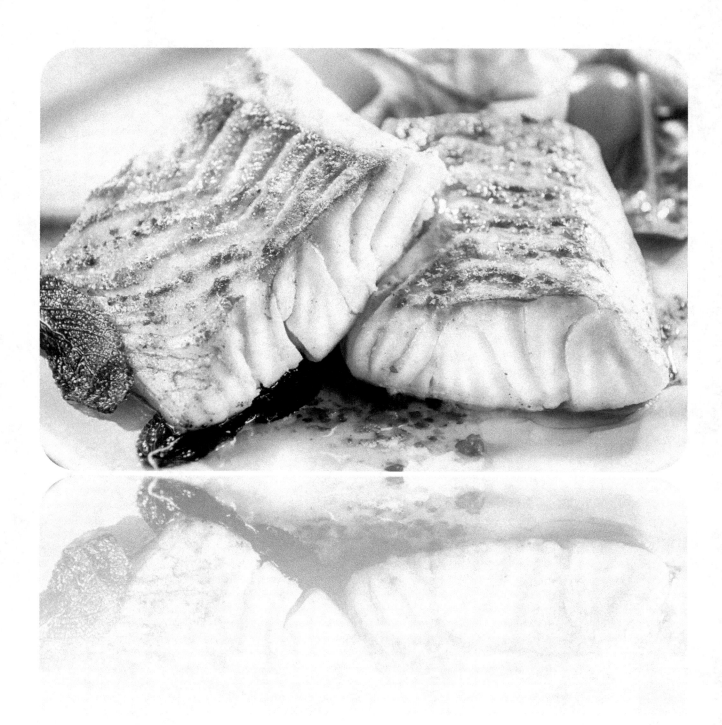

50. Blackened Catfish

Prep Time: 1 minute | Cooking Time: 40 minutes| Temperature: 450F|

Servings: 4

Ingredients:

Spice blend

- o 1 tsp. granulated garlic
- o 1/4 tsp. cayenne pepper
- o 1/2 cup Cajun seasoning
- o 1 tsp. ground thyme
- o 1 tsp. ground oregano
- o 1 tsp. onion powder

- o 1 tbsp. smoked paprika
- o 1 tsp. pepper

Fish

- o 4 catfish fillets
- o Salt to taste
- o 1/2 cup butter

Directions:

1. In a bowl, combine all the spice blend ingredients.
2. Sprinkle both sides of the fish with the salt and spice blend.
3. Preheat the grill to 450F.
4. Heat the cast iron pan and add the butter. Add the fillets to the pan.
5. Cook for 5 minutes per side.
6. Serve.

NUTRITION:

Calories: 181.5|Fat: 10.5g| Carb: 2.9g| Protein: 19.2g

51. Cajun Seasoning Shrimp

Prep Time: 10 minutes | Cooking Time: 16 to 20 minutes | Temperature: 400F | Servings: 4

Ingredients:

- 20 pieces of jumbo Shrimp
- 1/2 tsp. of Cajun seasoning
- 1 tbsp. of oil
- 1 tsp. of magic shrimp seasoning

Directions:

1. In a bowl, add oil, shrimp, and seasonings.
2. Mix well and coat the shrimps.
3. Put the shrimp on skewers.
4. Preheat the grill to 400F for 8 minutes.
5. Cook the shrimp for 2 minutes per side.
6. Serve.

NUTRITION:

Calories: 382|Fat: 7.4g| Carb: 23.9g| Protein: 50.2g

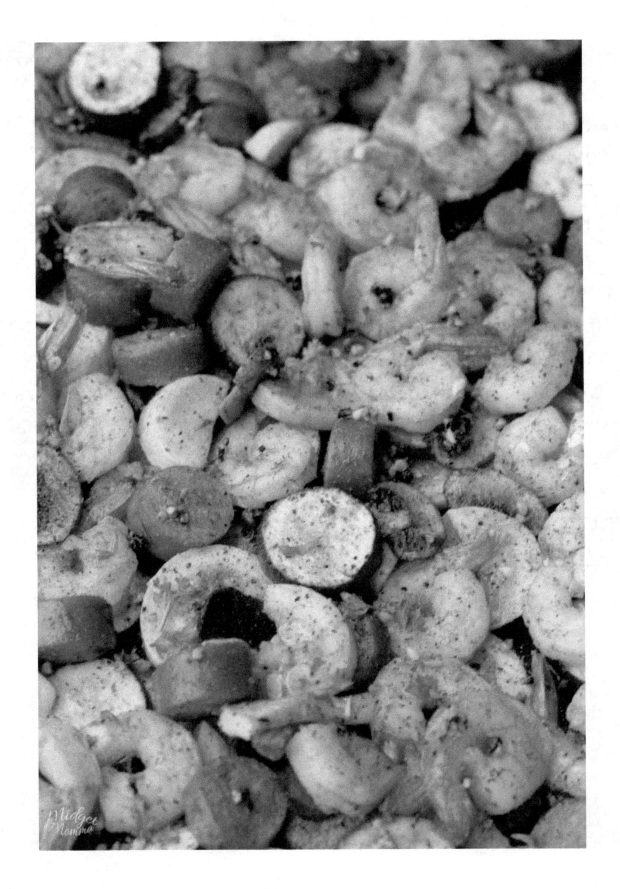

52. Juicy Smoked Salmon

Prep Time: 6 hours | Cooking Time: 50 minutes| Temperature: 220F| Servings: 5

Ingredients:

- ½ cup of sugar
- 2 tbsp. salt
- 2 tbsp. crushed red pepper flakes
- ½ cup fresh mint leaves, chopped
- ¼ cup brandy
- 1 (4 pounds) salmon, bones removed
- 2 cups alder wood pellets, soaked in water

Directions:

1. In a bowl, add brown sugar, crushed red pepper flakes, mint leaves, salt, and brandy, and make a paste.
2. Rub the paste all over your salmon and wrap the salmon with a plastic wrap.
3. Allow them to chill overnight.
4. Preheat, the smoker to 220F.
5. Smoke the salmon for 45 minutes or until flesh flakes off easily.
6. Serve.

NUTRITION:

Calories: 370|Fat: 8g| Carb: 1g| Protein:22g

53. Peppercorn Tuna Steaks

Prep Time: 8 hours| Cooking Time: 1 hour| Temperature: 250F|
Servings: 3

Ingredients:

- ¼ cup of salt
- 2 pounds yellowfin tuna
- ¼ cup Dijon mustard
- Freshly ground black pepper
- 2 tbsp. peppercorn

Directions:

1. In a large-sized container, dissolve salt in warm water (enough water to cover the fish).
2. Transfer tuna to the brine and cover, refrigerate for 8 hours.
3. Preheat the grill to 250F.
4. Remove tuna from bring and pat it dry.
5. Transfer to grill pan and spread Dijon mustard all over.
6. Season with paper and sprinkle peppercorn on top.
7. Transfer tuna to smoker and smoke for 1 hour.
8. Serve.

NUTRITION:

Calories: 307|Fat: 3g| Carb: 10g| Protein: 57

54. Jerk Shrimp

Prep Time: 15 minutes | Cooking Time: 6 minutes| Temperature: 450F|
Servings: 12

Ingredients:

- 2 pounds shrimp, peeled, deveined
- 3 tbsp. olive oil
- 1 tsp. garlic powder
- 1 tsp. of sea salt
- 1/4 tsp. ground cayenne
- 1 tbsp. brown sugar
- 1/8 tsp. smoked paprika
- 1 tbsp. smoked paprika
- 1/4 tsp. ground thyme
- 1 lime, zested

Directions:

1. Set the Traeger temperature to 450F and preheat for 5 minutes.
2. Meanwhile, mix all the spices in a bowl.
3. Place shrimp in a bowl and sprinkle with the prepared spice mix. Drizzle with oil and mix well.
4. Place shrimp on the grill grate and smoke for 3 minutes per side or until firm and cooked.
5. Serve.

NUTRITION:

Calories: 131|Fat: 4.3g| Carb: 0g| Protein: 22g

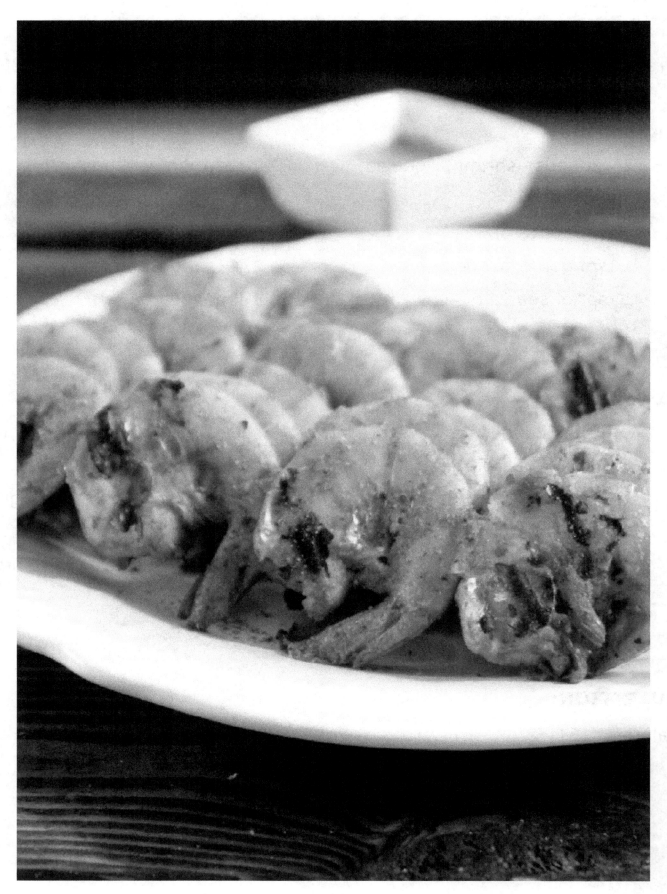

55. Lobster Tails

Prep Time: 10 minutes | Cooking Time: 35 minutes | Temperature: 450F| Servings: 4

Ingredients:

- 2 lobster tails, each about 10 ounces

For the Sauce:
- 2 tbsp. chopped parsley
- 1/4 tsp. garlic salt
- 1 tsp. paprika
- 1/4 tsp. ground black pepper
- 1/4 tsp. old bay seasoning
- 8 tbsp. butter, unsalted
- 2 tbsp. lemon juice

Directions:

1. Set the Traeger temperature to 450F and preheat for 15 minutes.
2. In a saucepan, add the butter and melt it. Add the remaining ingredients and mix well. Set aside.
3. To prepare the lobster – cut the shell from the middle of the tail, then take the meat from the shell, keeping it attached at the base of the tail. Butterfly the lobster tail.
4. Place lobster tails on a baking sheet, pour 1 tbsp. of sauce over each lobster tail and reserve the remaining sauce.
5. Place the tails on the grill grate and smoke for 30 minutes or until opaque.
6. Serve with the remaining sauce.

NUTRITION:

Calories: 290 |Fat: 22g| Carb: 1g| Protein: 20g

56. Lemon Garlic Scallops

Prep Time: 10 minutes | Cooking Time: 5 minutes| Temperature: 400F | Servings: 6

Ingredients:

- 1 dozen scallops
- 2 tbsp. chopped parsley
- Salt as needed
- 1 tbsp. olive oil
- 1 tbsp. butter, unsalted
- 1 tsp. lemon zest

For the Garlic Butter:

- ½ tsp. minced garlic
- 1 lemon, juiced
- 4 tbsp. butter, unsalted, melted

Directions:

1. Set the temperature of the grill to 400F and preheat for 15 minutes.
2. Season the scallops with salt and black pepper.
3. Place a skillet on the grill grate and add butter and oil. Place the seasoned scallops on the melted butter and cook for 2 minutes or until seared.
4. To make the garlic butter, take a small bowl, place all the ingredients, and whisk until combined.
5. Flip the scallops top with some prepared garlic bugger and cook for 1 minute more.
6. Transfer scallops to a dish, top with remaining garlic butter, sprinkle with parsley and lemon zest, and serve.

NUTRITION:

Calories: 184|Fat: 10g| Carb: 1g| Protein: 22g

57. Halibut in Parchment

Prep Time: 15 minutes | Cooking Time: 15 minutes | Temperature: 450F| Servings: 4

Ingredients:

- 16 asparagus spears, trimmed, sliced into 1/2-inch pieces
- 2 ears of corn kernels
- 4 ounces halibut fillets, pin bones removed
- 2 lemons, cut into 12 slices
- Salt as needed
- Ground black pepper as needed
- 2 tbsp. olive oil
- 2 tbsp. chopped parsley

Directions:

1. Set the Traeger temperature to 450F and preheat for 5 minutes.
2. Meanwhile, cut out 18-inch-long parchment paper, place a fillet in the center of each parchment, season with salt and black pepper, and then drizzle with oil.
3. Cover each fillet with three lemon slices, overlapping slightly, sprinkle ¼ of asparagus and corn on each fillet. Season with some salt and black pepper and seal the fillets and vegetables tightly to prevent steam from escaping the packet.
4. Place fillet packets on the grill grate and cover. Smoke for 15 minutes, or until packets have turned slightly brown and puffed up.
5. When done, transfer packets to a dish, let them stand for 5 minutes, then cut 'X' in the center of each packet, carefully uncover the fillets and vegetables. Sprinkle with parsley and serve.

NUTRITION:

Calories: 186.6|Fat: 2.8g| Carb: 14.2g| Protein: 25.7g

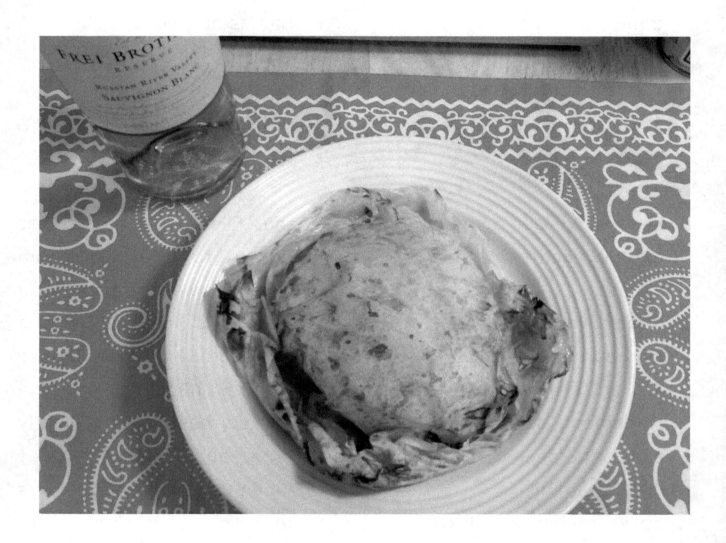

CONCLUSION

Traeger grill is a must-have outdoor kitchen appliance. This grill is revolutionary and has forever changed the way we cook. With new wood pellet grill series being produced each year, you need to shop smartly so that you buy a grill that perfectly fits you and meets all your needs. Whether you love grilling, smoking, roasting, or direct cooking of food, this versatile grill has got you covered. If you entertain guests regularly, then you do not have to worry because now you will be able to enjoy chit chats with them while your food is being grilled, thanks to the Traeger grill.

CPSIA information can be obtained
at www.ICGtesting.com
Printed in the USA
LVHW020730170621
690401LV00013B/808